ISBN No: 9781672182485

Preface:

This book is intended as a reference volume only, not as a medical manual or guide to self -treatment. If you suspect you have a medical problem, we urge you to seek competent medical help. Keep in mind that nutritional needs vary from person to person, depending on sex, age, health status, total diet. Information here is intended to help you make informed decisions about your diet and the nutritional and herbal supplements you choose, not to substitute for any treatment that may have been prescribed by your physician.

CONTENTS

VITAMINS

Introduction:

- Vitamins are organic molecules that are essential for normal healthy growth and development of body.

- Vitamins are non-caloric micronutrients that are needed in small amounts for normal body function.

- The "vita" part of the word "vitamin" means "life". They are vital and essential for life & health. Vitamins regulate metabolism & help in protects against diseases.

- optioned from food sourced like milk, fish, egg & green leafy vegetables etc.

Classification:

- Vitamins are classified according to how they are absorbed and stored in the body; vitamins are divided into two groups.

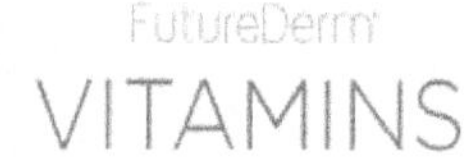

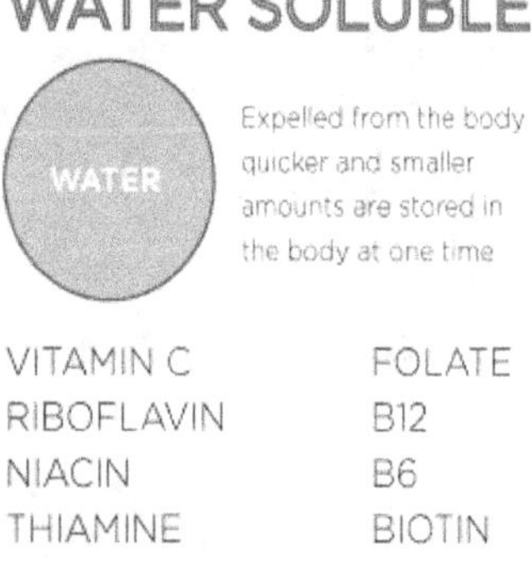

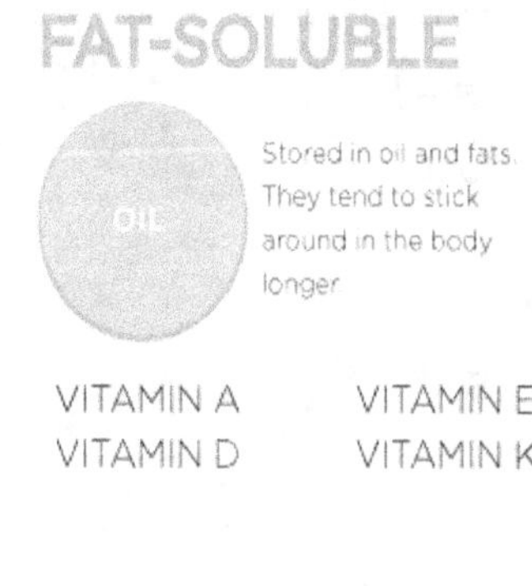

a) Fat-soluble vitamins: Includes vitamin A, D, E and K

- can be stored in the body, this storage usually occur in liver and fat tissue, storage decreases risk of deficiency, overconsumption can lead to toxicity; overconsumption from food is rare, it usually occurs from supplement.

b) **Water –soluble vitamins**: include vitamin C and B-complex vitamins.

- cannot be stored in body, except for B6 and B12, have no stable storage form and must be provided continuously in the diet.

- Vitamin B-complex is generally found in germinating seeds, wheat germ, pulses, beans and lentils, yeast, liver and meat. Bacteria of intestine mostly synthesize them. vitamin B-complex includes the seven B vitamins namely Thiamine (B1), Riboflavin (B2), niacin (B3), Pantothenic acid (B5), Pyridoxine (B6), Folic acid (B9), and cobalamine (B12) .

VITAMIN A: (Fat Soluble Vitamin)

The chemical name of Vitamin A is known as Retinol .Their parent substance is Beta-carotene, which is known as pro-vitamin. Vitamin A has major function in the Retina of the eye. Vitamin A is a fat soluble vitamin, have ability to travel through fat, restore in fat longer ,can go through cell wall because the layer of cells are made up of fat(lipid layers),while water soluble vitamin cannot.

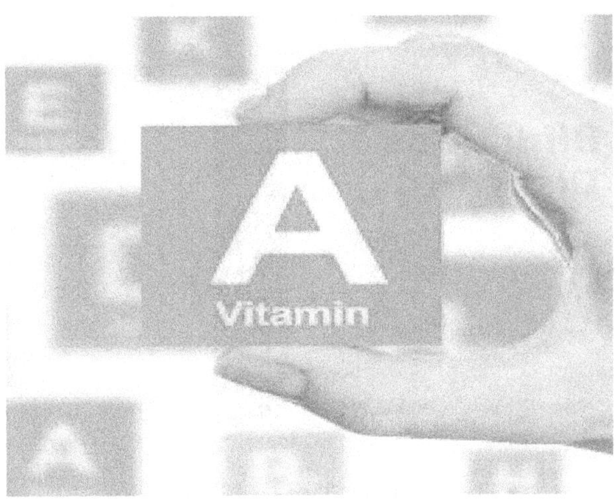

As Vitamin A is Fat-soluble, it is lost when milk is skimmed (when all the cream is removed from whole milk).In vegetables, Vitamin A exists as a Pro-vitamin in the form of Beta-carotene, which are yellow-orange pigments in the fruits and vegetables.

Function of Vitamin A:

- Vitamin A promotes normal vision.
- It is also required for the normal growth & Development of lacrimal glands (tear glands).

- Vitamin A maintains calcium levels in blood, promotes Growth & development of Bone, teeth, nerve and muscle function.
- It is necessary for reproduction.
- Vitamin A has anti- cancer property.
- Vitamin A act as anti-oxidants and prevents skin immune system.
- It is also essential for the maintenance of epithelial cells of skin and mucous membrane. Healthy epithelial cells do not allow infections, which is why vitamin A is also called as anti-infection vitamin.

Causes of vitamin A deficiency:

- Under nutrition mainly seen in developing countries due to poverty.
- Acute or Chronic infections generally seen in children.
- Malabsorption of fats, as vitamin A is fat soluble, possibly any damage in gut/digestive system occurs can lead to dryness of eyes and skin. Or the congestion of liver, unable to release bile to bile duct, which help in fat digestion.
- Therapeutic causes: Bariatric surgery, certain medications also inhibits the absorption of vitamin A.

Deficiency symptoms of vitamin A:

1. Changes in Eye

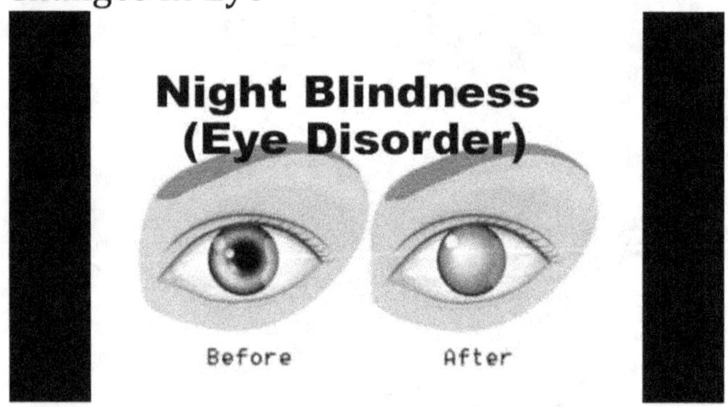

- Night blindness: (Nyctalopia) it is a condition making difficult or impossible to see in relatively low light/dim light, partial loss of vision/blurred vision.

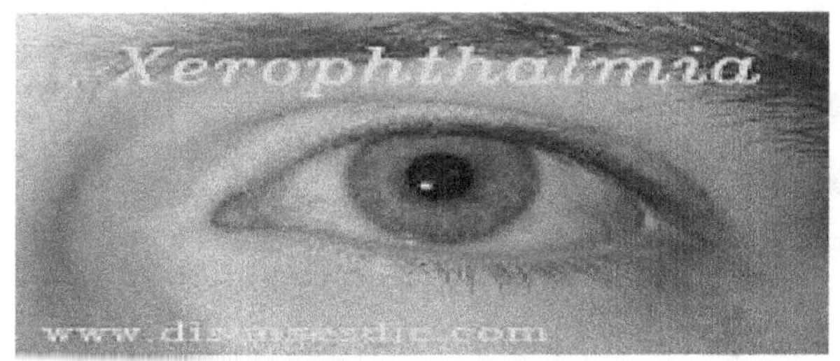

- Dryness of eye ball: (Xeropthalmia) Cornea becomes dry, wrinkled, lusterless, hazy and pigmented, tear glands stop secreting tears (mostly seen in pre-school (those age of 5 years) children's leading to corneal blindness.

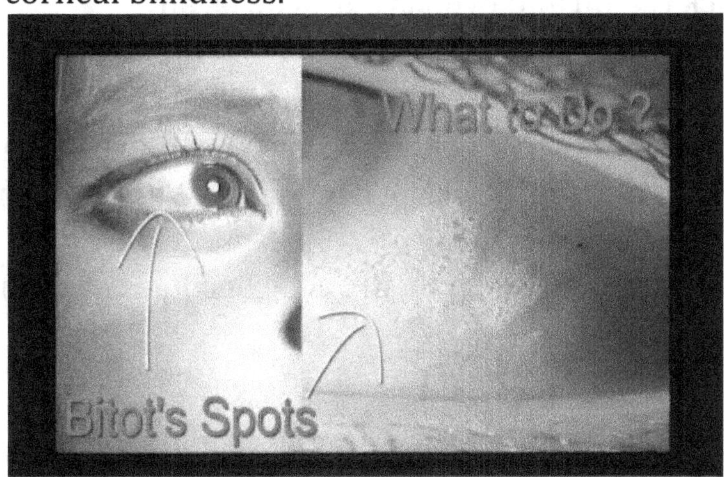

- Bitot spots: Clinical appearance: Small, Triangular, White patches resembling dried foam on the outer and inner sides of the cornea. Foamy appearance of bitot spots is due to gas production by coryne bacterium xerosis.
-

2. Changes in Skeletal system

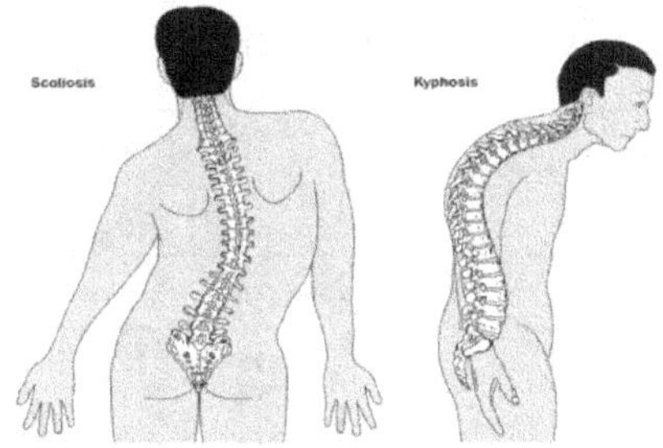

- Deficiency of Vitamin A leads to irregular development of skeleton (skull and vertebra), Reduce calcium in blood flow, more prone to fractures.

3. Changes in Skin

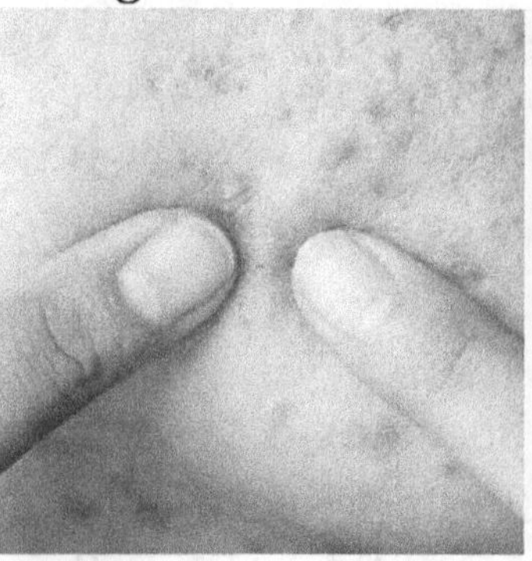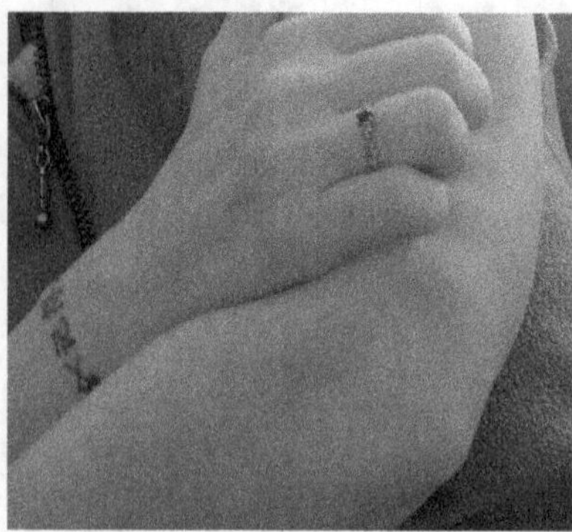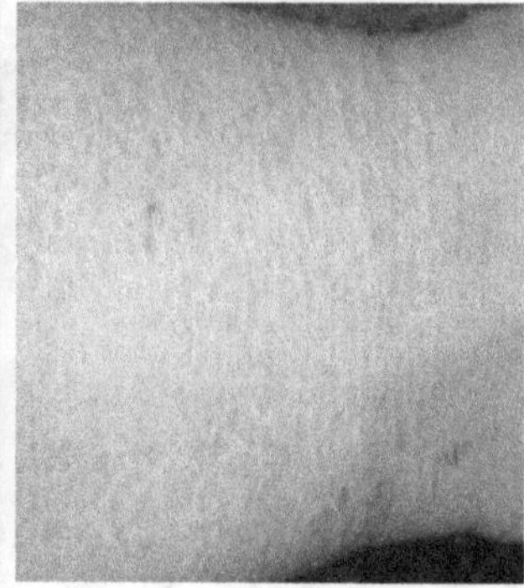

- Xeroderma : Skin becomes dry, Scaly with Itching, Different varieties of acne on face and back region and even cystic acne occur.

4. Changes in Respiratory Immunity

- Prone to more Infections, Specially in Children causing frequent Cough, Cold, Pneumonia, Tuberculosis(TB), Sinus, Ear & Lung Infections.
- Lining in the Nose, Throat, Trachea and Bronchi becomes dry and rough.

5. Changes in the Alimentary Canal/Digestive Tract

- Gets dried up which leads to Constipation, Lack of Absorption of Nutrients, Diminished secretion of digestive juices, More prone for Infection like Diarrhea

6. Pregnancy

- Specially more Vitamin A is required in Last 3 months before delivery, Otherwise the child may develop Night Blindness

Recommended Dietary Allowance (RDA) for Vitamin A

Age Groups	Particulars	Vitamin A (Beta-Carotene) per day
Infants	0-12 months	1.2 mg
Children	1-6 years	1.6 mg
	7-9 years	2.4 mg
Boys	10 -18 years	2.4 mg
Girls	10-18 years	2.4 mg
Man	Above 18 years	2.4 mg
Women	Above 18 years	2.4 mg
Pregnant Women	0-9 months	2.4 mg
Lactation	0-12 months	3.8 mg

Dietary Source of Vitamin A – Beta carotene

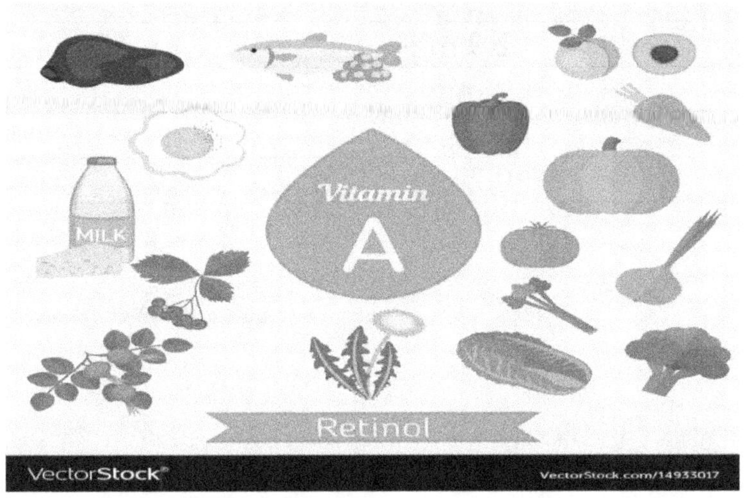

Green Leafy Vegetables	Vitamin A – Beta Carotene(mg per 100gm)
Drum stick leaves	19.7 mg
Methi/Fenugreek	9.2 mg
Amaranth leaves	8.6 mg
Curry leaves	7.1mg
Gogu leaves	5.8 mg
Chamakura aaku	5.5 mg
Onion leaf/ Ulliporaka	4.9 mg
Koyyala Kura	4.8 mg
Corriander leaves	4.8 mg
Pudina/Mint leaves	4.3 mg
Chennangiaku	11.9 mg
Mulla thota Kura	10.9 mg
Tulasi leaves	8.1 mg
Ponaganti kura	5.7 mg
Tummi kura	4.2 mg
Uttareni aaku	4.3 mg
Golimitti kura	1.9 mg

Tubers and Other vegetables	Beta carotene mg/100gm
Carrot	6.5mg
Sweet potato	1.8mg
Pumpkin	1.2 mg
Green Chillies	1 mg

Tomato ripe	0.6 mg

Fruits	Beta carotene mg/100gm
Dates	2.9 mg
Mango	2 mg
Papaya	1 mg
Orange	0.2 mg

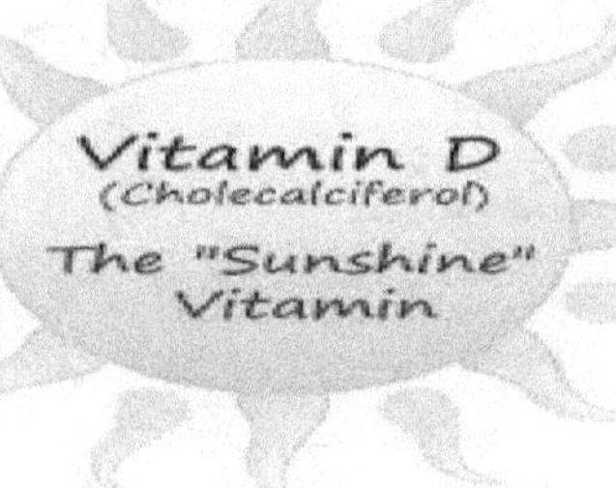

Functions:

- Promotes the absorption of calcium and phosphorous by the intestines, it affects the normal growth of the body and formation of teeth and bones.
- It maintains the normal functioning of parathormone (Harmones secreted by Parathyroid gland) which prevents the parathyroid gland towards suppressive acting of calcium
- Helps in regulation of cardio vascular system, renal system, Immune system, Central Nervous system, Reproductive organs, Skin, muscles and Bones.

Causes of Vitamin D Deficiency:

1. Chronic Kidney or Liver diseases can cause Vitamin D deficiency.
2. Calcium deficiency can also cause Vitamin D deficiency.
3. If melanin pigment is more (Dark skin), it also leads to Vitamin D deficiency.
4. Poor exposure to sun light.
5. Poor consumption of dairy.
6. Not Breast feeding in childhood.

<u>**Deficiency Symptoms**</u>:

Adults

1. Osteopenia : General bone and muscle pain, weak and fragile bone.

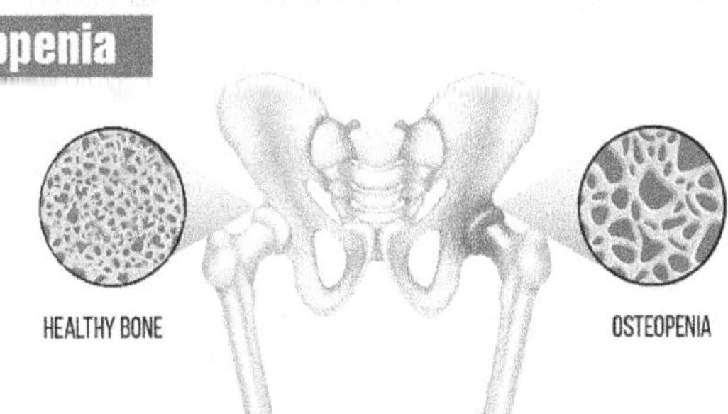

2. Osteomalasia : Painful condition due to poor mineralization of bones, Bones becomes extremely soft, fragile, deformed.

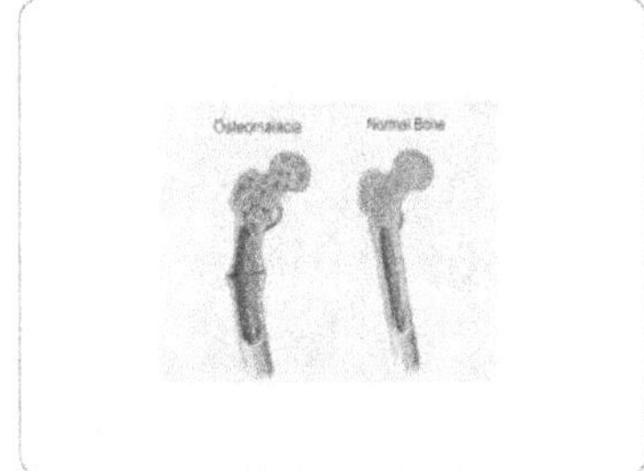

3. Dental caries: Cavities in teeth.

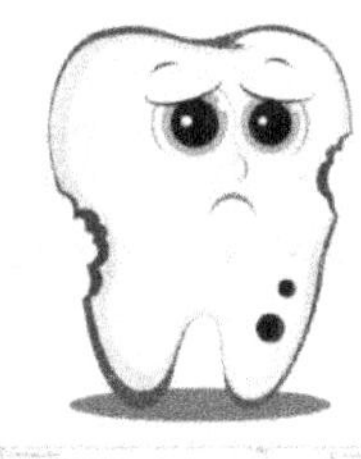

Children's

1. Rickets : Softness and Deformities of bones like Bow-legs and Pigeon chest

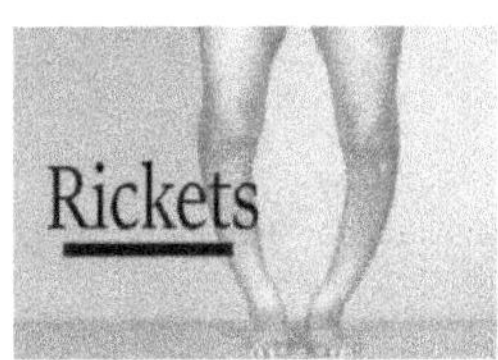

<u>**Recommended Dietary Allowance (RDA) for Vitamin D**</u>: For better calcium absorption, Is 10 mg / day for infants and growing children is required. In tropical countries with plenty of sunlight, smaller amount may sufficient. Adult's need less amount of vitamin D.

Dietary Source of Vitamin D:

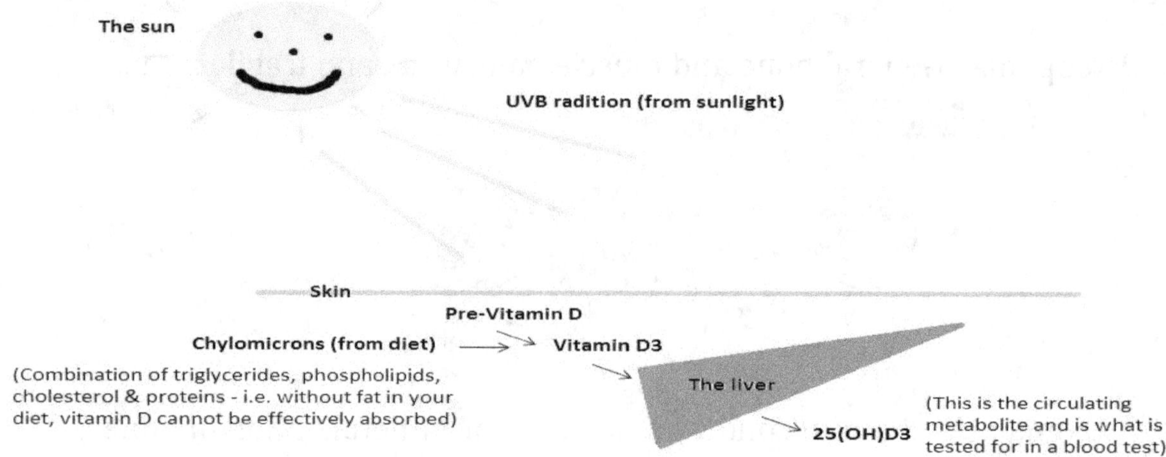

-Vitamin D is usually found in large quantities in the same foodstuffs, as vitamin A. Vitamin D is not actually a true vitamin because it is usually made in the body with the help of the sun's UV rays. The compound actually is actually made in the skin is a pro-hormone. Vitamin D does not act directly in the body. It is first converted into 25 hydroxy cholecalciferol in the liver and subsequently to 1,25-dihydroxy cholecalciferol (DHCC) in the kidney. 1, 25-DHCC is the active form of this vitamin D, which function in the body.

This vitamin is also formed in the skin by the UV rays present in sunlight, which converts a cholesterol derivatives β-dehydrocholesterol present in the skin to vitamin D.

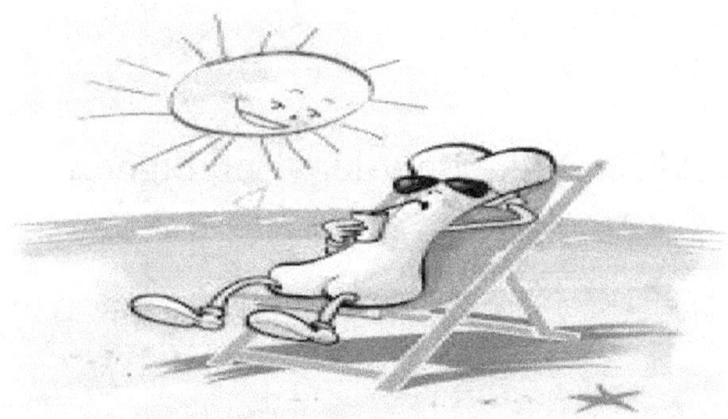

Note: To get a vitamin D from sunlight, the right time to expose to sunlight is between 11am-3pm the UV rays of sunlight at this time are more stronger, even early morning sunlight also give some amount of vitamin D,30% of the body should exposed to sunlight, for at list 15-20 minutes per day.

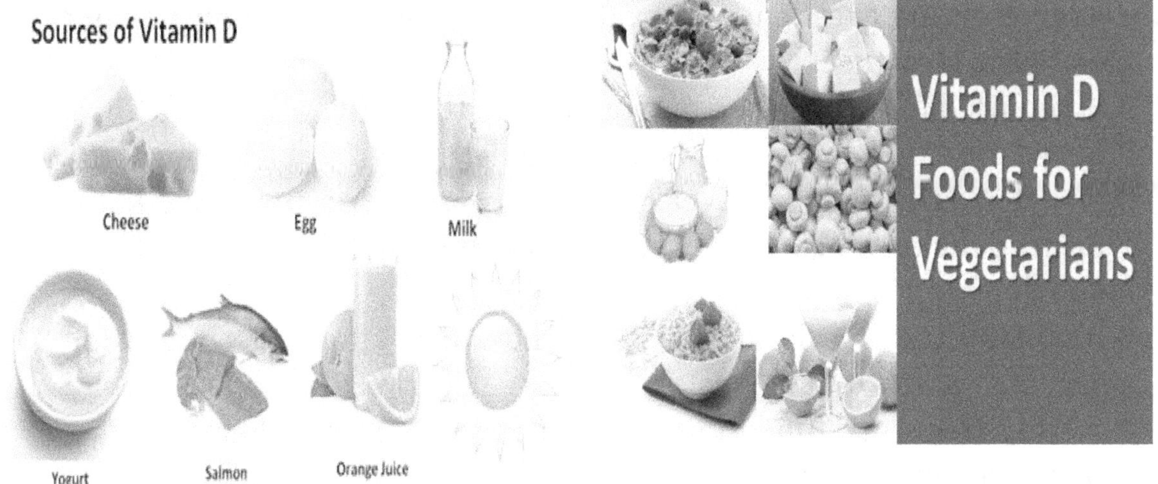

dietary source for vitamin D is : The highest amount of vitamin D is found in fish liver oil (e.g., cod liver oil)and other source are Milk , Curd, butter, cheese, egg yolk, white mushrooms (grown in sunlight), oranges, carrot, Pineapple.

The food grains (e.g., brown rice, Oats) grown in the sunlight has a trace amount of vitamin D in it.

The active form of vitamin E is known as Alpha-tocopherol

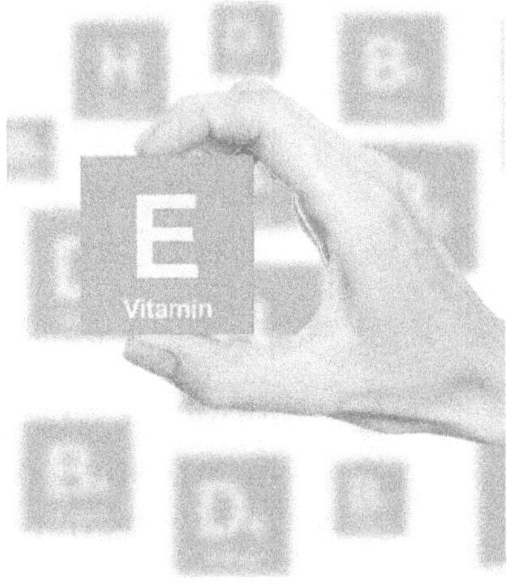

<u>**Functions:**</u>

- Tocopherols are excellent anti oxidants and thus maintain normal bio membrane structure.
- It is required for proper use of vitamin A in the body.
- It keeps the skin healthy, slows down aging.
- It also decreases fragility (Weakness) of the erythrocytes (RBC's), Thus its deficiency also causes Anemia in which RBC's are devoid of hemoglobin.
- It maintains the muscles of the body; Therefore, Vitamin E should be a part of athlete's diet.
- It maintains normal functioning of reproductive organs; hence it is called as fertility vitamin.
- It helps in development and cell formation. Thus it is needed in the diet of Pregnant, lactating women and for the new born infants, particularly premature infants.
- Vitamin E has anti cancer property. It is used for curing cancer
- It is also used to prevent heart attacks and treat an Alzheimer's disease in some patients.

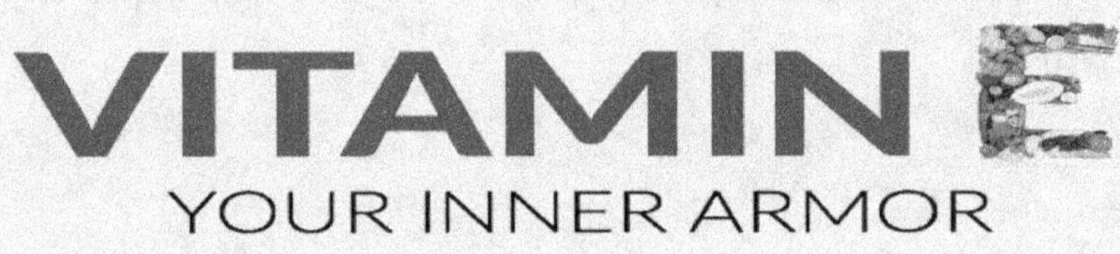

<u>**Deficiency Symptoms:**</u>

Particulars	Deficiency symptoms
Infants	- Weight Loss - Delayed growth - Poor eating habits - Physical and Mental developmental problems
Children's	- Muscle weakness - Loss of tendon movement reflux - Loss of postures senses - Slow growth - Motor speech disorder - Paralysis of eye movement

Adults	- Reproductive failure - Degeneration of muscles - Mild anemia (RBC's become fragile) - Non specific neurological defect - Slow growth and degeneration of the renal tubules - Exhaustion after light exercise - Slow wound healing - Lack of sex drive - Varicose veins and loss of muscle tone

Recommended Dietary Allowance (RDA) for Vitamin E

Male: 10 mg/day

Female: 8 mg/day

Pregnant and lactating: 15 mg/day

Dietary Source of Vitamin E

Green leafy vegetables	Vitamin E/100 gm
Curry leaves	1.71 mg
Spinach	1.27 mg
Pumpkin leaves	1.24 mg
Agathi leaves	1.48 mg

Grain legumes	Vitamin E/100 gm
Bengal gram, Whole	1.59 mg

Nuts and oil seeds	Vitamin E/100 gm
Pistachio nuts	31.41 mg
Safflower seeds	31.74 mg
Sun flower seeds	21.39 mg
Almonds	24.88 mg
Walnut	2.65 mg

Cashew nuts	1.05 mg
Coconut, Dry	6.02 mg
Coconut fresh	2.39 mg
Garden cress seeds	1.07 mg
Gingelly seeds, brown	1.24 mg
Ground nuts	4.26 mg
Mustard seeds	1.44 mg
Lin seeds/ Flax seeds	7.79 mg
Niger seeds, black	2.58 mg
Pine seeds	4.01 mg

Condiments and spices	Vitamin E/100 gm
Turmeric powder	2.63 mg
Poppy seeds	1.66 mg
Cumin seeds	1.49 mg
Nutmeg	1.18 mg
Mace	1.05 mg

Egg and Egg Products	Vitamin E/100 gm
Egg, poultry, whole, boiled	1.31 mg
Egg, poultry, omelet	1.82 mg

Vitamin K (Phylloquinone, Coagulation vitamin, Anti hemorrhagic vitamin)

Vitamin k is of two types

- Vitamin K1: This is abundant in vegetable oils, green leafy vegetables etc
- Vitamin K2: This is synthesized by the Intestinal bacteria
- *One cup of green tea made from leafs, provides a good amount of Vitamin K. As well as being an effective anti oxidant, green tea is a healthy alternative to tea or coffee.

Functions:

1. Blood coagulation: - Vitamin K is needed for the synthesis of blood clotting factor, prothrombin- Factor needed for the normal coagulator function of the blood.

2. Bone Metabolism: - Helps in bone healing and repair mechanism, it helps in production of bone protein osteocalcin, which is vital for the update of calcium and for maintaining bone mineral density.
3. It helps in preventing internal bleeding, hemorrhages and aids in reducing excessive menstrual flow.

Deficiency symptoms:

- Hemorrhage: Vitamin K deficiency resulting in faulty blood clotting and a increased tendency towards bleeding
- Bleeding on minor injuries- Fatal bleeding
- Internal bleeding- The extent of severity depends on bleeding rate and location of bleeding. Example: Heart, Brain, stomach & Lungs.
- Tenderness – Sensitivity to pain, sourness.

Causes of Vitamin K deficiency

- Do not take proper amount of green leafy vegetables
- Prolonged Exposure to Anti-microbial treatments
- Fat mal absorption, as vitamin K is fat soluble it is not absorbed well.

Recommended Dietary Allowance (RDA) for Vitamin K

0.07 – 0.14 mg/day

Dietary Source of Vitamin K

Cereals & Millets	Vitamin K/100 gm
Jowar	0.04 mg
Black gram	0.01 mg

Grains & Legumes	Vitamin K/100 gm
Field beans	0.02 mg
Green gram whole	0.01 mg
Horse gram	0.01 mg
Green peas, dry	0.01 mg
Red gram dal	0.04 mg
Red gram whole	0.09 mg

Green leafy vegetables	Vitamin K/100 gm
Ponnaganni kura	0.5 mg
Drum stick leaves	0.4 mg

Fenugreek leaves	0.4 mg
Gogu leaves	0.4 mg
Spinach	0.3 mg
Parsley	0.3 mg
Amaranth leaves	0.3 mg
Bathuna leaves	0.2 mg
Basella leaves	0.2 mg
Betel Leaves, big	0.2 mg
Pumpkin leaves	0.2 mg
Tamrind leaves	0.2 mg
Cabbage, green	0.1 mg
Cauliflower	0.1 mg

Other vegetables	Vitamin K/100 gm
Broad beans	0.09 mg
Pumpkin(orange color)	0.08 mg
Cucumber	0.07 mg
French beans	0.06 mg
Zucchini, yellow	0.05 mg
Onion	0.04 mg
Peas, fresh	0.04 mg
Capsicum, yellow	0.03 mg
Drum stick	0.03 mg
Cluster beans	0.02 mg
Field beans	0.02 mg
Jack fruit raw	0.02 mg
Ladies finger	0.02 mg
Tomato ripe	0.02 mg

Fruits	Vitamin K/100 gm
Custard apple	0.05 mg
Jack fruit	0.03 mg
Tamarind	0.03 mg
Pomegranate	0.01 mg
Strawberry	0.01 mg

Roots & Tubers	Vitamin K/100 gm
Lotus roots	0.04 mg
Carrot	0.01 mg

Condiments & Spices fresh	Vitamin K/100 gm
Green chillies	0.02 mg
Coriander leaves	0.2 mg
Curry leaves	0.2 mg
Ginger fresh	0.02 mg
Mint leaves	0.1 mg

Condiments & Spices – Dry	Vitamin K/100 gm
Red chillies	0.2 mg
Black pepper	0.1 mg
Cloves	0.1 mg
Cumin seeds	0.1 mg
Pippali	0.09 mg
Poppy seeds	0.09 mg
Mace	0.07 mg
Nutmeg	0.06 mg
Asofoetida	0.04 mg
Coriander seeds	0.03 mg
Omum	0.03 mg

Nuts & Oil seeds	Vitamin K/100 gm
Pine seeds	0.4 mg
Niger seeds	0.1 mg
Gingelly seeds	0.1 mg
Coconut fresh	0.02 mg

Vitamin C (Ascorbic Acid)

Functions:

- Vitamin C helps in formation of collagen, Bone matrix, Tooth denting and other extra cellular materials
- it is necessary for healthy gums and teeth
- It helps in the proper absorption and utilization of Iron in the body
- It helps in the production of anti bodies and for the formation of RBC's
- It helps in healing wounds and helps body to with stand Injury from burns and toxicity

- It has anti oxidant property
- It helps in metabolism of many acids by balancing the PH levels in the body
- Enhance the immune system of the body which protect us from cough and cold and stimulate
- It also helps to cure diabetes as Vitamin C helps in processing of Insulin and Glucose
- Reduce risk of stroke
- Reduce stress
- Prevents signs of aging
- Strengthen Skin, Hairs and Nails

Deficiency Symptoms:

- Lack of Vitamin C means that new collagen cannot be formed. This causes various tissues in your body start to break down, Health & Repair system of your body becomes affected.
- Persistent (Chronic) Vitamin C deficiency, usually over a period of around 3 months or more can leads to an illness known as scurvy.

Warning Signs of Vitamin C deficiency

- Slow wound healing
- Swollen, Bleeding and Inflamed gums
- Dry or splitting hair and nails
- Red, Rough, Dry skin
- Frequent Nose bleeding
- Swollen and painful joints
- Fatigue and Depression
- Un explained weight gain
- Poor immune function

Recommended Dietary Allowance (RDA) of Vitamin C

Particulars	Age groups	RDA of Vitamin C
Infants	0-12 months	25 mg/day
Children	1-18 years	40 mg/day
Male	Above 18 years	40 mg/day
Female	Above 18 years	40 mg/day

<u>**Dietary source**</u>:

Green leafy vegetables	Vitamin C / 100gms
Drum stick Leaves	108 mg
Ponnaganni	103 mg
Amaranth leaves	86 mg
Basella leaves	63.5 mg
Fenugreek leaves	58.2 mg
Raddish leaves	65.7 mg
Cabbage leaf	40.76 mg
Cauliflower leaf	40.71 mg
Beet green	35.83 mg
Gogu leaves	35.43 mg
Spinach	30.28 mg
Tamarind leaves	28.22 mg
Beetel leaves	25.51 mg

Other Vegetables	Vitamin C / 100gms
Capsicum, Green	127 mg
Mango raw	90.24 mg
Drum stick	71.86 mg
Cauliflower	47.14 mg
Bitter gourd	46.53 mg
Green peas fresh	38.4 mg
Tomato ripe	27.4 mg
Onion	27.2 mg
Ladies finger	22.5 mg
Papaya raw	20.73 mg

Fruits	Vitamin C / 100gms
Goosberry	252 mg
Guva	222 mg
Tamarind	55.78 mg
Star fruit	50.20 mg
Mango	49 mg
Lemon juice	48.16 mg
Sweet lime	46.9 mg
Papaya ripe	43.09 mg
Orange	42.72 mg
Pineapple	36.37 mg

Litchi	33.8 mg
Grape, seedless, black	27.32 mg
Wood aple	22.17 mg
Musk melon	22.76 mg
Custard apple	21.51 mg
Fig	16.92 mg
Jamun fruit	16.47 mg
Pomegranet, maroon seeds	12.69 mg

Roots and Tubers	Vitamin C / 100gms
Lotus root	26.63 mg
Potato, brown, small	26.41 mg
Potato, brown, big	23.15 mg
Sweet potato	22.20 mg

Condiments & Spices	Vitamin C / 100gms
Green chillies	100 mg
Coriander leaves	23.87 mg

B-Complex

Vitamin B1 (Thiamine):

Functions:

- Thiamine helps in the metabolism of glucose and production of energy
- It is essential for amino acid metabolism
- It plays an important role in tissue respiration, tones the nervous system and muscles, improves appetite and promotes growth
- It helps to reduce fatigue, stress, pain in muscles

Causative factors for Vitamin B1 deficiency:

- Consumption of polished rice, refined grains
- Stress, Difficulty in sleeping
- Alcohol, Liver damage(Fatty liver/Liver cirohosis)
- Usage of refines Carbohydrates and Sugars
- Women with extreme vomiting and nausea during pregnancy
- Usage of certain medications – Antiacids, Antibiotics, Diuretics, Pain killers

- Low stomach acid, Diarrhea
- Over usage of tea and coffee

Deficiency disorders:

1. Leads to berri berri
2. Tingling and numbness of hands and fingers, restless legs
3. Increases Heart rate, Edema
4. Dry cough at night times
5. Weakness in Nervous system

Recommended Dietary Allowance RDA for Vitamin B1

Particulars	Age groups	RDA for B1
Infants	0-12 months	0.5 mg
Children	1-3 years	0.6 mg
	4-6 years	0.9 mg
	7-9 years	1 mg
Boys	10-12 years	1.1 mg
	13-15 years	1.2 mg
	16-18 years	1.3 mg
Girls	10-18 years	1 mg
Men	Above 18 years	1.2 mg
Women	Above 18 years	1.2 mg

Dietary Source:

Thiamine occurs in the outer coats of seeds of many plants including the cereals grains. Unpolished rice and food made of whole grains are good source of vitamin B1. It is also synthesized by bacteria in the colon.

Cereals & Millets	Vitamin B1 / 100 gm
Wheat	0.46 mg
Raagi	0.37 mg
Barley	0.36 mg
Jowar	0.35 mg
Maize	0.33 mg
Varagu	0.29 mg
Brown rice	0.27 mg
Samelu	0.26 mg
Bajra	0.25 mg

Grains & Legumes	Vitamin B1 / 100 gm
Red gram, whole	0.74 mg
Green peas Dry	0.56 mg
Red gram, dal	0.45 mg
Green Gram, whole	0.45 mg
Bengal gram, whole	0.37 mg
Field beans	0.37 mg
Lentil dal	0.34 mg
Cow pea, brown	0.34 mg
Black gram, whole	0.32 mg
Horse gram	0.32 mg
Rajma	0.30 mg

Green leafy vegetables	Vitamin B1 / 100 gm
Spinach	0.16 mg
Gogu leaves	0.13 mg
Tamarind leaves	0.12 mg
Fenugreek leaves	0.11 mg

Other vegetables	Vitamin B1 / 100 gm
Broad beans	0.12 mg
Capsicum	0.14 mg
Baby corn	0.15 mg
Green peas	0.27 mg

Fruits	Vitamin B1 / 100 gm
Apricot, processed	0.25 mg

Nuts and Oil seeds	Vitamin B1 / 100 gm
Pistachio nuts	0.98 mg
Saff flower seeds	0.85 mg
Cashew nuts	0.61 mg
Sunflower seeds	0.59 mg
Ground nuts	0.57 mg
Mustard seeds	0.55 mg
Graden cress seeds	0.52 mg
Niger, Blackk	0.46 mg
Walnut	0.40 mg

Pine seeds	0.36 mg
Gingelly seeds, white	0.36 mg
Flax seeds	0.28 mg
Almonds	0.15 mg

Milk & Milk products	Vitamin B1 / 100 gm
Khoa	0.11 mg

Vitamin B2 (Riboflavin):

Functions:

- This vitamin is essential for growth & health.
- It maintains healthy skin & Oral mucosa.
- It helps in breakdown of carbohydrate, protein & fats. Essential for converting carbohydrate into energy.
- It also play important role in iron absorption, deficiency of vitamin B2 can lead to anemia.
- It is also associated with the physiology of vision.

Deficiency symptoms:

- Signs are mainly seen at mucocutaneous area (Pertaining to the mucous membrane & Skin). Mucocutaneous area of the body includes the mouth, eyes, vagina & Anus.
- Riboflavin deficiency results in poor growth & other pathological changes in skin, eyes, liver & nerves.
- Glossitis – Inflammation, painful &redness of the tongue, causes sourness with depapillation of the dorsal surface of the tongue, difficulty in chewing, swallowing or speaking.
- Cheilitis – Dry, cracked & pecling lips, inflammation of lips, allergic patches around your lips can cause due to frequent sun exposure.
- Angular stomatitis – The Corner of your mouth may be bleeding, red, swollen, cracked, blistered, crusty, itchy, scaly, painful condition is seen.
- Other symptoms include – Digestive disorders, burning sensation in the skin & eyes, racked heels, oily skin, eye redness, anal fissures, distance eye sight, migraine, mental depression, forgetfulness.

Recommended Dietary Allowance RDA for Vitamin B2

Particulars	Age groups	RDA for B2
Infants	0-12 months	0.06 mg
Children	1-3 years	0.6 mg
	4-6 years	0.9 mg
	7-9 years	1.0 mg
Boys	10-12 years	1.1 mg
	13-15 years	1.2 mg
	16-18 years	1.3 mg
Girls	10-18 years	1.0 mg
Men	Above 18 years	1.4 – 1.9 mg
Women	Above 18 years	1.1 – 1.5 mg

Dietary source:

Riboflavin is synthesized by green plants, mainly intestinal bacteria & fungi but not by animals. Certain dietary sources of Riboflavin are also known as Lactoflavin (from milk), Ovaflavin (from egg yolk), & Verdoflavin (from grass).

Cereals & Millets	Vitamin B2 / 100 gm
Wheat	0.46 mg
Bajra	0.20 mg
Barley	0.18 mg
Ragi	0.17 mg
Maize	0.12 mg

Grains & Legumes	Vitamin B2 / 100 gm
Red gram, whole	0.45 mg
Red gram, dal	0.45 mg
Green Gram, whole	0.45 mg
Bengal gram, dal	0.35 mg
Field beans	0.37 mg
Lentil dal	0.40 mg
Cow pea, brown	0.33 mg
Black gram, dal	0.32 mg
Horse gram	0.32 mg
Rajma	0.30 mg

Green leafy vegetables	Vitamin B2 / 100 gm
Drumstick leaves	0.45 mg

Fenugreek leaves	0.22 mg
Spinach	0.16 mg
Radish leaves	0.13 mg

Other vegetables	Vitamin B2 / 100 gm
Beans scarlet, tender	0.12 mg
Brinjal	0.11 mg

Condiments & Spices – fresh	Vitamin B2 / 100 gm
Garlic	0.20 mg
Green Chillies	0.11 mg

Condiments & Spices – dry	Vitamin B2 / 100 gm
Poppy seeds	0.87 mg
Asafoetida	0.82 mg
Cumin seeds	0.52 mg
Omum	0.30 mg
Fenugreek seeds	0.28 mg
Coriander seeds	0.19 mg
Mace	0.13 mg

Nuts and Oil seeds	Vitamin B2 / 100 gm
Niger,Gray	0.35 mg
Musturd seeds	0.33 mg
Almonds	0.26 mg
Niger, black	0.23 mg
Garden cress seeds	0.15 mg
Safflower seeds	0.15 mg
Sunflower seeds	0.13 mg
Walnut	0.12 mg
Gingelly seeds, black	0.10 mg
Cashew	0.03 mg

Miscellaneous	Vitamin B2 / 100 gm
Toddy	0.27 mg

Milk & Milk products	Vitamin B2 / 100 gm

Milk, Buffalo	0.13 mg
Milk, Cow (whole)	0.11 mg
Khoa	0.11 mg
Paneer	0.10 mg

Egg & Egg Products	Vitamin B2 / 100 gm
Egg Poultry, Whole omlet	0.20 mg
Egg Poultry, Whole boiled	0.18 mg

Functions:

- This vitamin is necessary for the metabolism of carbohydrates.
- It is also essential for the normal functioning of the gastrointestinal tract and the satisfactory functioning of the nervous system.
- It helps in treating high cholesterol by reducing triglyceride synthesis (inhibit lypolysis) basically it is helpful when lipid profile is getting altered, because it causes LDL(Low Density Lipoprotein), VLDL(Very Low Density Lipoprotein), Triglycerides, Bad Cholesterol to decrease. Therefore, it is used in the treatment of Hyper Lipidemia.
- It reduces the risk of stroke and heart attacks.
- It slows down the progress of the Type 1 Diabetes, cataracts.
- It reduces the risk of osteoarthritis, skin diseases, Alzheimer's disease.

NOTE: Niacin is a vitamin which is synthesized in the body with the help of an amino acid known as Tryptophan.

60 mg of Tryptophan is required to synthesis 1 mg of Niacin in body.

Causes of Niacin Deficiency:

- Popular group who consume the stale food like maze & Jowar, because it contain leucine which interference with the formation of Niacin. As leucine inhibits the Tryptophan absorption.
- Hartnup's disease, a hereditary abnormality in metabolism of Tryptophan is characterized by pellagra like skin rash, temporary ataxia (loss of the power of muscular coordination) and mental

deterioration. The urine of the patient of this disease contains increased amount of Tryptophan.
- Chronic Alcoholism reduces Niacin absorption.
- Deficiency of Riboflavin (B2), Pyridoxine (B6) & Iron, can also lead to Niacin Deficiency.

Deficiency symptom of Niacin:

- Deficiency of Niacin causes a disease called Pellagra (it is made up of an Italian word Pelle which means skin & agra means rough, pellagra = rough skin).
- It is characterized by four D's namely
    o Diarrhea – Watery stool.
    o Dermatitis – Inflammation of skin which becomes scaly and papillated (especially when skin is over exposed to sun light), Hyper pigmentation a thick flack like skin is seen around the neck is known as castel mean's neclase.
    o Dementia – Memory Loss, may also lead to madness, muscle atrophy and severe inflammation of mucous membrane of alimentary canal may occur.
    o Death – If pellagra is not treated well in time can also lead to death.

Recommended Dietary Allowance RDA for Vitamin B3

Particulars	Age groups	RDA for B3
Infants	0-12 months	0. 6 mg
Children	1-3 years	8 mg
	4-6 years	11 mg
	7-9 years	13 mg
Boys	10-12 years	15 mg
	13-15 years	16 mg
	16-18 years	17 mg
Girls	10-18 years	14 mg
Man	Above 18 years	16 – 21 mg
Woman	Above 18 years	12 – 16 mg

Dietary Source:

VitaminB3 (Niacin) is found in plant & animal tissues. Niacin can be formed in the body from the amino acid Tryptophan, which is present in all dietary proteins.

Cereals & Millets	Vitamin B3 / 100 gm
Brown rice	3.40 mg
Barley	2.84 mg
Maize	2.69 mg
Whole Wheat	2.68 mg
Single polished rice	2.51 mg
Wheat flour	2.37 mg
Jowar	2.10 mg
Puffed rice	1.87 mg
Rice flakes	1.60 mg
Raagi	1.34 mg
Samelu	1.29 mg
Wheat semolina	1.13 mg

Grains & Legumes	Vitamin B3 / 100 gm
Green peas, dry	2.69 mg
Lentil Dal, yellow	2.56 mg
Rajma, red	2.42 mg
Green gram, whole	2.16 mg
Bengal gram, whole	2.10 mg
Field beans, brown	2.04 mg
Black gram, whole	1.85 mg
Horse gram	1.82 mg
Cow pea, brown	1.64 mg

Green leafy vegetables	Vitamin B3 / 100 gm
Pumpkin leaves	1.49 mg
Garden cress leaves	1.20 mg
Agathi leaves	1.18 mg

Fruits	Vitamin B3 / 100 gm
Apricot, dried	1.66 mg
Tamrind pulp	1.56 mg
Dates, dry, brown	1.47 mg

Roots & Tubers	Vitamin B3 / 100 gm
Potato	1.36 mg

Condiments & Spices – fresh	Vitamin B3 / 100 gm
Green Chillies	1.06 mg

Condiments & Spices – dry	Vitamin B3 / 100 gm
Red Chillies	6.94 mg
Cumin seeds	2.87 mg
Turmeric powder	1.55 mg
Omum	1.23 mg
Coriander seeds	1.20 mg
Fenugreek seeds	1.19 mg
Cloves	1.15 mg
Cardamom, green	1.13 mg
Pippali	1.06 mg

Nuts and Oil seeds	Vitamin B3 / 100 gm
Ground nuts	11.35 mg
Garden cress seeds	5.67 mg
Mustard seeds	3.80 mg
Almonds	3.71 mg
Pine seeds	3.52 mg
Gingelly seeds	3.12 mg
Sunflower seeds	1.60 mg
Niger seeds	1.14 mg
Safflower seeds	1.12 mg
Lin seeds	1.09 mg
Cashew nuts	1.03 mg

Vitamin B5 (Pantothenic acid): Anti graying factor, Anti stress factor

Functions:

- This vitamin is good for skin & Hair. It prevents from allergy & strengthens immune system.
- It is required for the normal functioning of adrenal gland. It helps adrenal gland to properly produce cortisol (stress harmones), which fight against Inflammations.
- Vitamin B5 helps to reduce accumulation of Lactic acid in the body. Pain after exercise occurs due to lactic acid accumulation.

- Vitamin B5 allows to use carbohydrates, proteins & fat for energy.
- It helps in lowering the levels of cholesterol & Triglycerides.
- It helps in fast wound healing (especially after surgery.)
- Prevents rheumatoid arthritis.

Deficiency symptoms of Vitamin B5:

People develop Vitamin B5 deficiency when they are chronicle in stress, & even people suffering from urinary tract infection.

- A classic sign of vitamin B5 is Burning foot syndrome "Burning feet Neuropathy"
- Adrenal fatigue
- Insomnia, Fatigue, Depression.
- Head ache, Irritability.
- Stomach pain, Vomiting.
- Grey Hair, Acne.

Recommended Dietary Allowance RDA for Vitamin B5: Is About 5 – 15 mg per day.

Dietary source:

The word pantothenic in Greek language means "from everywhere". Hence, it is widely distributed and is found in various foods like Cereals & Millets, Grains & Legumes, Fruits, Nuts & Oil seeds, Milk & Egg etc., Usually B5 deficiency is not seen because it is present in all veggies.

Vitamin B6:

Functions:

- The vitamin B6 helps in the metabolism of Amino acids (Protein Metabolism).
- Vitamin B6 Pyridoxine helps in the generation of the Niacin B3 from Tryptophan & thus B6 deficiency can also cause pellagra.
- Vitamin B6 is useful in the treatment of Nausea & Vomiting during Pregnancy (Morning sickness), Muscular dystrophy & radiation sickness.
- It also maintains nervous system by helping in mylenation of nerves.
- It acts as catalyst mainly in glycogen break down, if sugar cells problem in blood sugars.

Causative factors for deficiency of Vitamin B6:

- Over consumption of Alcohol.
- Any damage or dysfunction in Liver.
- Leaky gut or any type of Irritable bowel syndrome.
- Insulin resistance is seen in Type 2 Diabetes.
- Rheumatoid arthritis.
- Over usage of antibiotics, steroids & oral contraceptives.

Deficiency symptoms of Vitamin B6:

- Dermatitis, Cracked corner mouth.
- Nausea, Vomiting, Fatigue, Tiredness.
- Neuropathy, Convulsion (Fits), Sleep Apnea, Unable to wakeup.
- Type 2 Diabetes.
- Fluid Retention.
- Carple tunnel syndrome, Trigger finger.

Recommended Dietary Allowance RDA for Vitamin B6

Particulars	Age groups	RDA for B6
Infants	0-6 months	0.1 mg
	6 – 12 months	0.4 mg
Children	1-3 years	0.9 mg
	4-6 years	0.9 mg
	7-9 years	1.6 mg
Boys	10-12 years	1.6 mg
	13-15 years	2.0 mg
	16-18 years	2.0 mg
Girls	10-12 years	1.6 mg
	13-18 years	2.0 mg
Man	Above 18 years	2.0 mg
Woman	Above 18 years	2.0 mg
Pregnant Woman	0-9 months	2.5 mg
Lactation	0-12 months	2.5 mg

Dietary Source:

Cereals & Millets	Vitamin B6 / 100 gm
Maize	0.45 mg
Brown rice	0.37 mg
Amaranth seeds(Rajgira)	0.33 mg

Barley	0.31 mg

Grains & Legumes	Vitamin B6 / 100 gm
Black gram, whole	0.53 mg
Lentil whole, Brown	0.46 mg
Red gram, whole	0.42 mg
Bengal gram, whole	0.36 mg
Green gram, whole	0.35 mg

Green leafy vegetables	Vitamin B6 / 100 gm
Drumstick leaves	0.87 mg
Fenugreek leaves	0.38 mg
Gogu leaves	0.33 mg

Other vegetables	Vitamin B6 / 100 gm
Bean scarlet, tender	0.31 mg
Ladies Finger	0.27 mg
Capsium	0.25 mg
Green peas	0.19 mg
Onion	0.17 mg
Green mango	0.13 mg
Drumstick	0.12 mg

Fruits	Vitamin B6 / 100 gm
Banana, ripe	0.44 mg
Pomegranate	0.29 mg
Gooseberry	0.27 mg
Jack fruit	0.22 mg
Raisins, Black	0.17 mg
Water melon	0.17 mg
Guava	0.16 mg
Fig(Anjeer)	0.15 mg
Dates, Dry	0.14 mg
Pine apple	0.13 mg

Roots & Tubers	Vitamin B6 / 100 gm
Yam, Elephant	0.22 mg

Lotus roots	0.19 mg
Carrot	0.11 mg
Potato	0.10 mg

Condiments & Spices	Vitamin B6 / 100 gm
Garlic	0.77 mg
Curry leaves	0.57 mg
Chillies, green	0.45 mg
Ginger, fresh	0.20 mg
Coriander leaves	0.19 mg
Mint leaves	0.17 mg
Onion	0.12 mg

Condiments & Spices Dry	Vitamin B6 / 100 gm
Fenugreek seeds	0.77 mg
Pipalli	0.66 mg
Poppy seeds	0.42 mg
Red chillies	0.42 mg
Cumin seeds	0.39 mg

Nuts & Oil seeds	Vitamin B6 / 100 gm
Pistachio nuts	0.96 mg
Sunflower seeds	0.94 mg
Saff flower seeds	0.93 mg
Walnuts	0.80 mg
Gingelly	0.49 mg
Niger seeds	0.45 mg

Sugars	Vitamin B6 / 100 gm
Jaggery	0.71 mg
Sugarcane, juice	0.40 mg

Vitamin B9 (Folic acid, Folate)

Functions:

1. Prevention of birth defects (specially defects of Brain/Spinal cord)
2. Reduce risk of coronary heart disease

3. Also important for the growth and formation of RBC's, Prevents anemia
4. It helps in DNA synthesis
5. Prevents from Depression, Dementia, Alzheimers cognitive function
6. Folic acid reduce the risk of cancers (Breast, Survical, Colon, Pancreatic & Stomach)

<u>Deficiency symptoms</u>:

1. Anemia (Pale skin)
2. Chronic low energy, Change in mood, Irritability, Headache
3. Premature Hair graying, Poor growth
4. Mouth Ulcers, Peptic ulcers (Inflammation of intestines), Diarrhea, Poor digestion (Inability to absorb, specially fats)
5. Glossitis- Swollen tongue, Sour or Tender mouth.

<u>Causes for Folic acid deficiency</u>:

- Alcohol consumption.
- Pregnancy, Morning sickness.
- Eating food which is over cooked or poor in nutrition.
- Liver & Kidney metabolic disorders.
- Mal absorption – Celiac disease.

<u>Recommended Dietary Allowance RDA of Folic Acid</u>:

Particulars	Age groups	RDA for B9
Infants	0-12 months	0.02 mg
		0.4 mg
Children	1-3 years	0.03 mg
	4-6 years	0.04 mg
	7-9 years	0.06 mg
Boys	10-12 years	0.07 mg
	13-15 years	0.10 mg
	16-18 years	0.10 mg
Girls	10-12 years	0.07 mg
	13-18 years	0.10 mg
Man	Above 18 years	0.10 mg
Woman	Above 18 years	0.10 mg
Pregnant Woman	0-9 months	0.40 mg
Lactation	0-12 months	0.40 mg

<u>**Dietary sources:**</u>

Cereals & Millets	Vitamin B9 / 100 gm
Varagi	0.039 mg
Jowar	0.039 mg
Samai	0.036 mg
Bajra	0.036 mg
Raagi	0.034 mg
Wheat	0.030 mg

Grains & Legumes	Vitamin B9 / 100 gm
Rajmah	0.33 mg
Field beans	0.29 mg
Cow pea	0.24 mg
Bengal gram	0.23 mg
Red gram	0.22 mg
Horse gram	0.16 mg
Green gram	0.14 mg
Black gram	0.13 mg
Peas, dry	0.11 mg

Green leafy vegetables	Vitamin B9 / 100 gm
Spinach	0.14 mg
Agathi (Avise akulu)	0.12 mg
Tamarind leaves	0.09 mg
Gogu leaves, red	0.08 mg
Amaranth, red	0.08 mg
Fenugreek leaves	0.07 mg
Drumstick leaves	0.04 mg
Cabbage	0.04 mg
Cauliflower	0.04 mg

Other vegetables	Vitamin B9 / 100 gm
Field beans, tender, broad	0.12 mg
Bitter guard	0.06 mg
French beans	0.06 mg
Drumstick	0.06 mg
Ladies finger	0.06 mg
Capsicum	0.05 mg

Jack fruit seeds	0.05 mg
Green peas, fresh	0.05 mg
Onion	0.05 mg
Bottle guard	0.04 mg
Brinjal	0.03 mg

Fruits	Vitamin B9 / 100 gm
Mango	0.08 mg
Papaya, ripe	0.06 mg
Avocado	0.06 mg
Bael fruit	0.05 mg
Pomegranate, Maroon	0.03 mg
Raisins, black	0.03 mg
Guava	0.03 mg
Jack fruit	0.03 mg

Roots & Tubers	Vitamin B9 / 100 gm
Beetroot	0.09 mg
Radish	0.02 mg
Carrot	0.02 mg

Condiments & Spices fresh	Vitamin B9 / 100 gm
Curry Leaves	0.17 mg
Mint leaves	0.10 mg
Garlic	0.08 mg
Coriander leaves	0.05 mg
Onion	0.02 mg

Condiments & Spices dry	Vitamin B9 / 100 gm
Poppy seeds	0.07 mg
Nutmeg	0.07 mg
Pippali	0.06 mg
Omum	0.05 mg
Fenugreek seeds	0.05 mg
Red chilies	0.05 mg

Nuts & Oil seeds	Vitamin B9 / 100 gm
Niger seeds	0.14 mg

Gingelly seeds	0.12 mg
Groundnut	0.09 mg
Mustard seeds	0.09 mg
Lin seeds	0.08 mg
Safflower seeds	0.08 mg
Sunflower seeds	0.08 mg
Walnut seeds	0.05 mg

Sugars	Vitamin B9 / 100 gm
Sugar cane juice	0.04 mg

Milk & Milk products	Vitamin B9 / 100 gm
Paneer	0.09 mg
Khoa	0.09 mg

Egg & Egg products	Vitamin B9 / 100 gm
Boiled egg, whole	0.11 mg

Vitamin B12 (Cyanocobalmin):

Water soluble vitamins except vitamin B12 have no stable storage form & must be provided continuously in the diet. Vitamin B12 can be stored in the liver.

Function:

- Vitamin B12 plays an important role in the synthesis of nucleic acid (Base of DNA).
- It stimulates the bone marrow to produce RBC's. Thus it is important for the formation & maturation of RBC's.
- Vitamin B12 is required for maintenance of energy, brain function & many others.
- Vitamin B12 plays an important role in detoxification function.
- It helps to make fuel for Muscle cell & helps to develop neurons.

Causes of Vitamin B12 deficiency:

- The absorption of B12 requires intrinsic factor, which is (produced along with stomach acid) intrinsic factor is a glucoprotein made in the stomach along with HCL which helps the B12 to get absorbed.

- For genetic reasons, some people do not make intrinsic factor lead to B12 deficiency(even they take supplements also)
- With age, the stomach makes less acid – less intrinsic factors. Prone to more Vitamin B12 deficiency.
- Pre menopausal women develop B12 deficiency.
- Certain medications also inhibit the absorption of Vitamin B12, Drugs which inhibits the secretion of stomach acid like antacids, antihistamines, etc.

Deficiency symptoms:

- Deficiency of Vitamin B12 leads to pernicious anemia (greater decrease in the number of RBC's formation in the bone marrow). Pernicious anemia refers to a type of auto immune anemia which causes a fall in the number of red blood cells. Leads to weakness, tiredness, fatigue, vertigo.
- Vitamin B12 is required for RBC formation in the presence of intrinsic factors secreted by stomach lining. If the secretion of the intrinsic factor stops, its deficiency disturbers normal synthesis of nucleic acids particularly DNA.
- Its deficiency also causes nervous disorders like fatigue, tiredness, mood swings, irritability, tingling of nerves, and numbness in hands & legs in sleep, memory loss, confusion and sleep apnea.
- Depression (Reversible with B12 supplements)
- Greater risk of cardiovascular disease & cancer.
- Other symptoms like Heart palpitation, pale skin shortness of breath, smooth tongue, burning sensation, constipation, Frequent gastric issue, loss of appetite & taste.
- Loss of vision, loss of weight, hyper thyroid, loss of muscle strength.
- Skin leasons, unexplained skin health issues, hyper pigmentation.

Recommended Dietary Allowance RDA of Vitamin B-12.

Particulars	Age groups	RDA for B12
Infants	0-12 months	0.2 µg
Children	1-9 years	0.2 µg – 1.0 µg
Boys	10-18 years	0.2 µg – 1.0 µg
Girls	10-18 years	0.2 µg – 1.0 µg
Man	Above 18 years	1 µg
Woman	Above 18 years	1 µg
Pregnant woman	0-9 months	1 µg

| Lactation | 0-12 months | 1.5 µg |

Dietary sources:

Vitamin B12 is a dark red compound containing cobalt. It is not found in plants. Strict vegetarians may be at risk of B12 deficiency. Poultry, meat, fish are good source of this vitamin. It is also synthesized by intestinal bacteria, which in fact are main source of Vitamin B12.

- Milk (250 ml of milk contains 1.4 µg of vitamin B12) & Milk products such as curd, paneer, cheese.
- Almond milk, coconut milk.
- Mushrooms.
- Egg (Boiled egg, whole / omelet).
- All fruits & Vegetables (Balanced Diet).
- Orange Juice.
- Soya products (soya nuggets, tofu).
- Cereals- brown rice.

MINERALS

Introduction:

Minerals are inorganic chemical elements that the body needs for healthy growth & metabolism. They are involved in making harmones & enzymes. If minerals are not present in the proper proportion, then vitamins are not sufficiently absorbed. Our body needs them in trace to small amounts. Helps regulates body function such as assisting the muscle contraction & regulating the enzyme activities.

Nearly all minerals are best absorbed in there free form except Iron.

General functions of Minerals elements:

- Minerals are necessary for the formation of blood & bone. Body fluids, cellular growth & Healing, energy, muscle tone & nerve function.
- All elements work together as a collective whole. A deficiency of one mineral may disturb the entire chain of life; the balance of the entire bodily activity can be thrown away.
- All nutrients such as Vitamins, Proteins, Enzymes, Amino Acids, Carbohydrates, Fats, Sugar etc., require minerals for their proper activity.
- The body must maintain an adequate mineral supply to maintain cell function.
- Hormonal secretion is dependent upon mineral stimulation.
- Acid – Alkaline balance (pH) of Tissue fluid is controlled by minerals.

Minerals are divided into three main categories:

a) **Macro Minerals:** These minerals are required in large amount at least 100 mg per day like Calcium, Phosphorus, Sodium, Chlorine & Potassium.

b) **Micro Minerals:** These minerals are required in less amounts, generally less than 100 mg per day like Magnesium, Manganese, Iron, Sulphur, Boron etc.,

c) **Trace Minerals:** These minerals are required in few micro grams including Zinc, Iodine and Fluorine.

Calcium

The body contains more calcium than any other minerals. 99% of the total calcium is concentrated in the bones & teeth; the remaining is in the fluids & soft tissues. Calcium is an essential element for living organisms, is required for normal growth & development. Calcium is absorbed from the food through the walls of intestine; this process is helped with the presence of Vitamin D.

Functions of Calcium:

- Calcium is required for the proper growth & development of healthy bones, teeth, gums & nails strength.
- It helps to maintain optimal body weight & ensures healthy alkaline pH levels.
- It improves immunity of the body
- Calcium controls nerves & muscles excitability & Nerve impulses.
- Calcium aids in blood clotting, controls cholesterol level & blood pressure, protect cardiac muscle.
- Calcium aids in transportation of nutrients in body.
- Calcium helps in B12 absorption & reduces menstrual cramps, prevent pre menstrual depression.
- During pregnancy calcium is required for proper growth & development of fetus.
- Calcium reduces the risk of colon cancer.

Causative factors for Calcium deficiency:

- Calcium deficiency is rare but can occur when there is lack of vitamin D or problem with absorption through the intestinal walls.
- Low dietary intake
- Mal-absorption due to low stomach acid, celiac disease.
- High intake of wheat brain, phosphates, animal fats.
- Lactose intolerance
- Usage of the contraceptive pill, corticosteroid drugs, diuretic drugs.
- Pregnancy – repeated pregnancies coupled with inadequate dietary intake can also give rise to calcium deficiency.
- Brest feeding less than one year.

Deficiency symptoms of Calcium:

- Deficiency of Calcium can leads to conditions such as rickets in children (Symptoms include delayed growth, bow legs, weakness and pain in the spine, pelvis and legs) & osteomalacia in adults.
- Rickets in childhood if not treated may encourage the development of osteoporosis in later life.
- Calcium deficiency leads to weaken bones, teeth, nails & hair.
- Other deficiency symptoms are bone pain, joint pain, fragile bone, arthritis / rheumatoid arthritis, muscle weakness & cramps delayed in healing of bone fractures, increased in muscle spasms & twitches (calf muscle spasms in sleep), tooth decay, brittle nails, nervousness, insomnia, high blood pressure.
- Calcium deficiency leads to osteoporosis in post menopausal woman.

Supplementation of Calcium rich food is required in following conditions:

a) **Osteoporosis:** Demineralization of bone leads to weak & brittle bones, increase risk towards fractures.
b) **Hypothyroidism:** The condition in which body don't generate enough calcium, and your body experience deficiency of calcium.
c) **Premenstrual syndrome:** By the consumption of calcium rich foods during this period reduces the symptoms up to 50% in woman experiencing head ache, moodiness, food craving, bloating, menstrual cramps these all occur due to Calcium deficiency.
d) **Cardio vascular disease:** Reduce the risk of heart attack by reducing the cholesterol levels.

Recommended Dietary Allowance RDA of Calcium:

Particulars	Age groups	RDA for Ca
Infants	0-12 months	500 mg
Children	1-9 years	400 mg
Boys	10-15 years	600 mg
	16-18 years	500 mg
Girls	10-15 years	600 mg
	16-18 years	500 mg
Man	Above 18 years	400 mg
Woman	Above 18 years	400 mg
Pregnant Woman	0-9 months	1000 mg
Lactation	0-12 months	1000 mg

<u>**Dietary sources:**</u>

Cereals & Millets	Calcium / 100 gm
Amaranth seeds	181 mg
Raagi	364 mg

Grains and Legumes	Calcium / 100 gm
Horse gram	269 mg
Soya beans	239 mg
Rice brain	200 mg
Mothbean	154 mg
Bengal gram	150 mg
Red gram	139 mg
Rajmah	134 mg
Green gram	92.4 mg
Black gram	86 mg
Cowpea	81 mg

Green leafy vegetables	Calcium / 100 gm
Agathi leaves (Avise akulu)	901 mg
Ponnaganni leaves	388 mg
Amaranth Leaves	330 mg
Drum stick leaves	314 mg
Fenugreek leaves	274 mg
Pumpkin leaves	271 mg
Radish leaves	234 mg
Garden cress leaves	217 mg
Bathua leaves	211 mg
Betal leaves	207 mg
Mustard leaves	191 mg
Cabbage, green	170 mg
Beet green	151 mg
Gogu leaves	145 mg
Spinach	82 mg
Tamarind leaves	66 mg

Other vegetables	Calcium / 100 gm
Cluster beans	121 mg
Ladies finger	86.12 mg

Field beans	70 mg
Broad beans	64.3 mg

Fruits	Calcium / 100 gm
Tamarind pulp	149 MG
Fig	78.5 mg
Raisins, dried, black	73.2 mg
Dates, dry, brown	71.2 mg

Condiments & Spices – fresh	Calcium / 100 gm
Curry leaves	659 mg
Mint leaves	205 mg
Coriander leaves	146 mg

Condiments & Spices – dry	Calcium / 100 gm
Poppy seeds	1372 mg
Omum	1032 mg
Cumin seeds	878 mg
Coriander seeds	718 mg
Clove	567 mg
Pippali	414 mg
Pepper	405 mg
Cardamom	378 mg
Asafetida	266 mg
Fenugreek seeds	135 mg

Nuts & Oil seeds	Calcium / 100 gm
Gingelly seeds, black	1664 mg
Gingelly seeds, white	1283 mg
Niger seeds, black	572 mg
Mustard seeds	403 mg
Garden cress seeds	318 mg
Lin seeds	257 mg
Almonds	228 mg
Safflower seeds	211mg
Sunflower seeds	176 mg
Pistachio nuts	135 mg
Walnut	105 mg

Sugars	Calcium / 100 gm
Jaggery	107 mg

Milk & Milk Products	Calcium / 100 gm
Koha	602 mg
Paneer	476 mg
Milk, whole, buffalo	121 mg
Milk, whole, cow	118 mg

Egg & Egg products	Calcium / 100 gm
Poultry, yolk, boiled	120 mg
Poultry, whole, boiled	55.2 mg

IRON

Iron is an important trace mineral that is found in every cell of the body, it usually combine with protein. Iron is essential mineral for human because it is a part of human blood cell. The major portion of it is found in blood as hemoglobin. Muscle tissue contains of about 3% of iron & the rest is stored in the liver, spleen, kidney & bone marrow.

Functions of Iron:

- One of the most important functions of iron is to make the protein called hemoglobin, hemoglobin is present in RBCs and helps to carry oxygen from lungs to rest of our body
- Iron transport oxygen & carbon-dioxide to & from cells.
- Iron helps to convert food into energy.
- Iron helps in synthesis of ATP. Mainly bringing about the oxidative changes within the tissues.
- There is a small amount of iron in the plasma. In the case of iron deficiency in the blood, the level of plasma iron comes down & Anemia occurs.
- Iron is present in the muscles as myoglobin. Myoglobin is a respiratory pigment present in the muscles of vertebrates & invertebrates. Myoglobin has a capacity of storing the oxygen in the muscles for the use in muscle contraction.

Source of Iron:

Absorption of iron mainly depends upon it source. Iron occurs in two forms in foods, as Haem Iron & Non-Haem Iron.

- Haem Iron – found in other animal protein.
- Non-Haem Iron – found in both plants & animal derived food.

Essential nutrients that help in iron absorption:

Iron requires Calcium, Vitamin C & other micro nutrients like manganese, copper; zinc for the absorption of the iron from the diet as the above minerals helps to capture the non Haem iron and stores it in a form that more easily absorb by your body.

Deficiency symptoms of Iron:

- Fatigue & tiredness.
- Shortness of breath.
- Dull & pale skin.
- Hair loss, brittle nails,
- Frequent head ache, leg pains, muscle cramps & soreness.
- Dullness & Depression.
- Increase sensitivity to cold.

Causes of Deficiency:

- Low dietary intake of iron rich foods.
- Malabsorption due to lack of stomach acid.
- Deficiency in woman is mainly seen due to menorrhagia, heavy bleeding.

Recommended Dietary Allowance RDA of Iron:

Particulars	Age groups	RDA for Fe
Infants	0-12 months	-
Children	1-3 years	12 mg
	4-6 years	18 mg
	7-9 years	26 mg
Boys	10-12 years	34 mg
	13-15 years	41 mg
	16-18 years	50 mg
Girls	10-12 years	19 mg
	13-15 years	28 mg

	16-18 years	30 mg
Man	Above 18 years	28 mg
Woman	Above 18 years	30 mg
Pregnant Woman	0-9 months	38 mg
Lactation	0-12 months	30 mg

Dietary Source:

Cereals & Millets	Iron / 100 gm
Amaranth seeds	9.3 mg
Bajra	6.42 mg
Raagi	4.62 mg
Rice, puffed	4.55 mg
Wheat flour	4.1 mg
Jowar	3.95 mg
Varagu	2.3 mg

Grains and Legumes	Iron / 100 gm
Horse gram	8.76 mg
Soya beans	8.29 mg
Mothbean	7.91 mg
Lentil whole	7.91 mg
Lentil dal	7.06 mg
Bengal gram, whole	6.78 mg
Bengal gram, dal	6.08 mg
Rajmah	6.30 mg
Black gram, dal	5.97 mg
Cow pea	5.90 mg
Field beans	5.50 mg
Green gram	4.89 mg
Peas, dry	5.09 mg
Red gram	3.9 mg

Green leafy vegetables	Iron / 100 gm
Gogu leaves, Red	9.56 mg
Gogu leaves, Green	7.65 mg
Amranth leaves, red	7.25 mg
Garden cress seeds	6.19 mg
Beet grecn	5.80 mg

Fenugreek leaves	5.69 mg
Pumpkin leaves, tender	5.58 mg
Parsley	5.51 mg
Ponnaganna	3.88 mg
Radish leaves	3.82 mg

Other vegetables	Iron / 100 gm
Cluster beans	3.90 mg
Onion, stalk	3.09 mg
Green peas, fresh	1.58 mg
Field beans, tender, broad	1.48 mg

Fruits	Iron / 100 gm
Tamarind pulp	9.16 mg
Raisins, dry, black	6.81 mg
Raisins, dry, golden	4.26 mg
Dates, dry, brown	4.79 mg
Dates, dry, pale brown	3.20 mg
Apricot, dried	2.50 mg
Gooseberry	1.25 mg

Roots & Tubers	Iron / 100 gm
Lotus roots	3.34 mg
Yam, elephant	1.22 mg

Condiments & Spices – fresh	Iron / 100 gm
Curry leaves	8.67 mg
Mint leaves	8.56 mg
Coriander leaves	5.30 mg

Condiments & Spices – dry	Iron / 100 gm
Turmeric powder	46.08 mg
Poppy seeds	10.13 mg
Mace	22.69 mg
Omum	13.65 mg
Cumin seeds	20.58 mg
Coriander seeds	17.64 mg

Clove	9.41 mg
Pippali	7.99 mg
Pepper	11.91 mg
Cardamom	8.33 mg
Asafetida	15.68 mg
Fenugreek seeds	8.47 mg
Red chilles	6.23 mg

Nuts & Oil seeds	Iron / 100 gm
Gingelly seeds, black	13.90 mg
Gingelly seeds, white	15.04 mg
Niger seeds, black	19.61 mg
Mustard seeds	13.49 mg
Garden cress seeds	17.20 mg
Lin seeds	5.44 mg
Almonds	4.59 mg
Safflower seeds	4.06 mg
Sunflower seeds	5.85 mg
Pistachio nuts	4.50 mg
Walnut	3.21 mg
Ground nuts	3.44 mg
Cashew nuts	5.95 mg
Pine seeds	4.50 mg

Sugars	Iron / 100 gm
Jaggery, cane	4.63 mg

Egg & Egg products	Iron / 100 gm
Poultry, yolk, boiled	4.92 mg
Poultry, whole, boiled	1.87 mg

Zinc

Zinc is a vital trace mineral that is required for a healthy-immune and DNA repair. Trace of zinc is found in all body tissue. The highest concentration of it occurs in the liver, Pancreas, Kidney and brain. It is also present in red blood cells and blood serum.

Functions of Zinc:

- Numerous aspect of cellular metabolism is Zinc- dependent. Approximately 300 different enzymes are dependent on zinc with their ability to do vital chemical reactions.
- Zinc plays an important role in growth and development, Boost immune response, neurological functions & reproduction.
- Zinc plays an important role in the formation of structure of protein and cell membrane. Loss of zinc from cell increases its susceptibility towards oxidative damage and impairs their function.
- Zinc plays an important role in Hormone release and nerve impulse transmission.
- Zinc is also essential for bone growth, sexual development, maintenance of blood sugar levels (zinc is essential for insulin production)
- Zinc is required for the absorption of vitamin A, B6 and iron.
- Helps to Maintains acid-alkaline (pH) balance in the body.
- Zinc is essential mineral to maintain health of Prostate, ovaries and testes.

Deficiency symptoms:

- Poor immune system, falling ill more frequently.
- Slowing or cessation of growth of nails and hair.
- Skin shows pimples, cystic acne, skin rashes, premature aging.
- Delayed sexual maturation, behavioral disturbances(depression, stress)
- Characteristic skin rashes, increase in hair fall.
- Impaired wound healing
- Diminished appetite, impaired smell & taste sensation.

Causes of Zinc deficiency:

- High intake of refined/processed foods.
- Alcoholism
- Iron supplement reduce the absorption of zinc.

- Hormonal imbalance, oestrogen also affects zinc levels.
- Contraceptive pill causes a drop in zinc.

Recommended Dietary Allowance RDA of Zinc: Is 8 -11 mg per day.

Dietary sources:

Zinc is present in most foods both of vegetable & of animal origin, but the richest sources tend to be protein-rich foods such as meat, seafood's & eggs. Most zinc comes from cereal grains and legumes.

Cereals & Millets	Zinc / 100 gm
Amaranth seeds	2.52 mg
Bajra	2.76 mg
Raagi	2.53 mg
Rice, puffed	1.45 mg
Wheat flour, atta	2.85 mg
Jowar	1.96 mg
Varagu	1.65 mg
Samai	1.82 mg
Brown rice	1.68 mg
Barley	1.50 mg
Rice flakes	1.49 mg
Wheat, semolina	2.13 mg

Grains and Legumes	Zinc / 100 gm
Horse gram	2.71 mg
Soya beans	4.01 mg
Lentil whole, yellow	3.31 mg
Lentil dal	3.61 mg
Bengal gram, whole	3.37 mg
Bengal gram, dal	3.65 mg
Rajmah	3.08 mg
Black gram, dal	3.0 mg
Cow pea	3.41 mg
Field beans	2.44 mg
Green gram	2.49 mg
Peas, dry	3.10 mg
Red gram	2.99 mg

Nuts & Oil seeds	Zinc / 100 gm
Gingelly seeds, black	8.59 mg
Gingelly seeds, white	7.84 mg
Niger seeds, black	4.98 mg
Mustard seeds	4.03 mg
Garden cress seeds	4.83 mg
Lin seeds	4.86 mg
Almonds	3.50 mg
Safflower seeds	3.90 mg
Sunflower seeds	7.07 mg
Pistachio nuts	2.42 mg
Walnut	2.94 mg
Ground nuts	3.18 mg
Cashew nuts	5.34 mg
Pine seeds	4.18 mg

Egg & Egg products	Zinc / 100 gm
Poultry, yolk, boiled	3.59 mg
Poultry, whole, boiled	1.31 mg

Selenium

It's an important mineral for immune system required in trace amounts. It is an important mineral for human health.

Functions of Selenium:

- It is best known as an antioxidants (repair damaged cell & DNA).
- It acts as catalyst for the production & maintenance of thyroid. It has anti inflammatory property.
- Selenium is required for support to reproduction, reduce the risk of miscarriages.
- It reduces the risk of heart disease, atherosclerosis (by lowering cholesterol levels).
- Helps to maintain normal function of liver, eyes, hair & skin.
- It acts as a key nutrient in counter acting the development of virus in the body (HIV).
- It protects the body against toxic metabolites & cancer cells growth.

Deficiency symptoms:

- Infertility in Men.
- Reduce immunity & resistance to infections.
- Causes inflammations of muscles.
- Impaired growth of the cells.
- Impaired production of active thyroid hormone.
- Increasing risk towards heart diseases, cataract, Arthritis, Cancer.

Causes of Deficiency:

- High intake of refined/ processed foods.
- High intake of foods grown on selenium deficient soil, Selenium absorption largely dependent on the soil it was grown in.

Recommended Dietary Allowance RDA of Selenium: Is 0.2- 0.4 mg per day.

Dietary sources:

Selenium can be found in some sea foods & meat. Plant source of selenium depends upon the plants that were grown in selenium-rich soil have higher levels of selenium in their muscles. Some of nuts & oil seeds are also a good source of selenium. Food rich in selenium :-

Niger seeds – 0.15 mg, Mustard seeds – 0.07 mg, Lin seeds – 0.04 mg, Garden cress seeds – 0.05 mg, Omum – 0.08 mg, Beet green – 0.04 mg, Lentil dal – 0.05 mg, Wheat – 0.05 mg.

Potassium

Potassium is an essential nutrient which controls the electric potential of the nervous system. 99% of total potassium present in body is found in cells. The remaining is distributed in the extra cellular fluid of the body. Some amount of potassium is also present in plasma. Potassium can be easily absorbed from the stomach & intestine. It is also present in digestive juices in large amounts. Excess potassium is excreted out from the kidney. Potassium is closely related to sodium, often it work along with it, but to opposite effect.

Potassium & sodium together controls the electrical potential of the nervous system, allowing signals to transmit & muscle to contract regularly.

Functions of Potassium:

- The most important electrolyte. To regulate levels of fluids in the body.
- It places a major role in maintaining the salt & water balance in the body & in maintaining optimal osmotic pressure within the body cells.
- Potassium is crucial in establishing the appropriate pH of blood.
- Potassium assists in the contraction of the muscles of the body as well as leading to effective working.
- Potassium is required for the proper working of nervous system, muscles & the heart (prevent cardiac arrhythmia).
- Potassium prevents from occurrence of stroke in human brain. By helping deliver oxygen to the brain.
- Potassium reduces the osteoporosis in woman.
- It helps in secretion of insulin for blood sugar control.
- It also stimulates peristalsis movement of food through digestive track.

Causes of deficiency:

- Kidney malfunction can cause potassium deficiency.
- Diet high in fat, refined sugars & over salted foods may quickly leads to a state of potassium deficiency.
- Vomiting, Diarrhea, Excess water loss, high cholesterol, diabetes.
- Lack of Magnesium leads to potassium deficiency.

Deficiency symptoms:

- Can leads to muscle weakness, cramps, fatigue, thirst, constipation, bloating, loss of appetite, problem with kidney & nervous system.
- Increases insulin level, Increases sugar craving.
- Abnormal heart beat, high blood pressure, insomnia.

Recommended Dietary Allowance RDA of potassium: Is 1600 - 2000 mg per day.

Cereals & Millets	potassium / 100 gm
Amaranth seeds	413mg
Bajra	365 mg
Raagi	443 mg
Wheat flour, atta	311 mg

Grains and Legumes	Potassium / 100 gm
Horse gram	1065 mg
Soya beans	1613 mg
Lentil whole, yellow	764mg
Lentil dal	786 mg
Bengal gram, whole	935mg
Bengal gram, dal	957 mg
Rajmah	1324 mg
Black gram, dal	1157 mg
Cow pea	1241 mg
Field beans	1272 mg
Green gram	1177 mg
Peas, dry	922 mg
Red gram	1303 mg

Green leafy vegetables	Potassium / 100 gm
Spinach	625 mg
Amranth leaves, red	564 mg
Betel leaves	678 mg
Beet green	530 mg
Agathi leaves	674 mg

Other vegetables	Potassium / 100 gm
Bitter guard	326 mg
Brinjal	302 mg
Cauliflower	329 mg
Drum sticks	419 mg
Field beans	520 mg

Fruits	Potassium / 100 gm
Avocado	377 mg
Bael fruit	409 mg
Banana, ripe	362 mg
Dates, dry, Pale brown	804 mg
Dates, dry, Dark brown	782 mg
Muskmelon, orange	206 mg
Pomegranate, maroon seeds	206 mg
Peach	281 mg
Raisins, dried, black	1105 mg

Raisins, dried, golden	913 mg
Tamarind pulp	816 mg

Roots & Tubers	Potassium / 100 gm
Lotus roots	611 mg
Yam, elephant	501 mg
Sweet potato	345 mg
Potato	541 mg
Beet root	306 mg

Condiments & Spices – fresh	Potassium / 100 gm
Curry leaves	584 mg
Mint leaves	539 mg
Coriander leaves	546 mg

Condiments & Spices – dry	Potassium / 100 gm
Turmeric powder	2374 mg
Poppy seeds	646 mg
Mace	623 mg
Omum	1692 mg
Cumin seeds	1886 mg
Coriander seeds	1473 mg
Clove	1434 mg
Pippali	1852 mg
Pepper	1487 mg
Cardamom	1262 mg
Fenugreek seeds	891 mg
Red chilles	2245 mg

Nuts & Oil seeds	Potassium / 100 gm
Gingelly seeds, black	480 mg
Gingelly seeds, white	491 mg
Niger seeds, black	716 mg
Mustard seeds	694 mg
Garden cress seeds	952 mg
Lin seeds	655 mg
Almonds	699 mg
Safflower seeds	550 mg

Sunflower seeds	559 mg
Pistachio nuts	1053 mg
Walnut	457 mg
Ground nuts	679 mg
Cashew nuts	635 mg
Pine seeds	686 mg

Sugars	Potassium / 100 gm
Jaggery, cane	458 mg

Sodium

Sodium is present in many foods in the form of sodium-chloride. 50% of total sodium present in body is found in extra cellular fluid & remaining is seen in bone, blood plasma & intracellular fluid. The absorption of sodium chloride occurs in the gastro-intestinal tract rapidly. The kidney regulates the sodium level in the body. Then the sodium levels in the body becomes excess is excreted through kidney.

Function of sodium:

- Sodium ions are the main ions in the fluid contained in the cells of the body.
- The interaction between the sodium & potassium ions is essential for survival & normal functioning of nerves & muscles.
- Sodium regulates water-salt balance in the body & maintains the acid alkaline balance (balance the pH level of body).
- Sodium play an important role in manufacturing of adrenaline (a hormone secreted by the adrenal gland) and amino acids (protein).
- Your body needs sodium to regulate blood pressure & ensure that your nerve cells & muscles work properly.

Deficiency symptoms:

- If sodium levels have dropped below normal level leads to a condition such as weakness, headache, nausea, vomiting, low appetite, confusion, irritability, restlessness, fatigue & low energy, muscular cramps & spasm.
- Sodium deficiency causes Electrolyte imbalance.
- Sodium deficiency includes internal gases, weight loss, poor memory, low blood sugar, heart palpitation.

<u>**Causes of Deficiency**</u>:

- Condition such as diarrhea, dehydration, liver disease, heart problem and even hypothyroidism can cause sodium levels to drop below normal.
- Loss of water through sweat occurs due to hard exercise or work can also leads to dehydration.
- Frequent exposure to the diuretic drugs can also leads to sodium deficiency.
- Sodium loss is more in addisons disease (deficiency of adrenal hormone)

<u>**Excess of sodium (hypernatraemia)**</u>:

- Too much of sodium can rise the blood pressure, and makes the blood pressure worse in people who are already suffering from hyper tension.
- It can also lead to cardiac failure and nephritis.
- It can also cause migraine head ache, mental confusion, fluid retention.
- Estrogen hormone favors sodium retention, which leads to oedema (swellings in the body) before the onset of menstruation & during pregnancy.
- If it is not corrected initially it can also leads to seizures & even comma.

<u>**Recommended Dietary Allowance RDA of sodium**</u>: Is 8-10 gm of sodium (sodium chloride/ salt) is required per day, is sufficient for an average adult. However our body adjusts to excess sodium intake.

<u>**Dietary source**</u>:

- Sodium deficiency is very rare because most foods contain some amount of sodium.
- The most common form of sodium is sodium chloride which is table salt.
- Drinking water also contains some amount of sodium; it varies depending upon the source.

Magnesium

Magnesium is an element which is stored in the body cell, primarily in bones & muscles. 30 – 40% of the available magnesium is taken up/

absorbed in to the blood stream through the intestines. The percentage of absorption increases if there is less magnesium in blood stream. The amount of magnesium present in the body is less than the amount of calcium & Phosphorous. If calcium intake increases the requirement of magnesium also increases. The unabsorbed magnesium is excreted from Urine & feces.

Functions of Magnesium:

Magnesium is an essential element which is required for the proper functioning if the body in many ways.

- Magnesium is required for the functions of nerves, muscles, immune & cellular system of the body.
- Magnesium is a co-factor for hundreds of enzymes is a helper factor that helps for metabolism of energy, protein (hair, nail, skin & muscle).
- Magnesium play important role in absorption of Vitamin B12 and calcium.
- It helps to reduce stress, headache, sleep apnea, Insulin resistance.
- It helps in strengthening of bones & teeth, promotes healthy muscles by helping them to relax.
- Beneficial for post menopausal woman, by strengthening heart muscles &nervous system.

Deficiency Symptoms:

- In deficiency of magnesium muscles become weak, the person feels fatigued & may develop irregular heart beat.
- It can also leads to development of kidney stones (due excess calcium in the body)
- Deficiency of magnesium leads to decreases of the potassium from the cell wall and that being replaced by sodium & calcium.
- The communication between the nerve cells & muscle function decreases in magnesium deficiency.
- Shortage of magnesium can gradually develop the symptoms like anxiety, fatigue, muscle weakness, cramps, insomnia, restless legs, and nausea.

Causes of Magnesium deficiency:

- A deficiency of magnesium may result from Malabsorption syndrome, chronic alcoholism and toxemia (blood poisoning by toxins from a local bacterial infection) of pregnancy or intake of diuretics.
- Low dietary intake – eating more refined foods and lack of green leafy vegetables.

Recommended Dietary Allowance RDA of Magnesium:

Particulars	Age groups	RDA for Magnesium
Man	Above 18 years	400-420 mg/ day
Woman	Above 18 years	310-320 mg/ day

<u>Dietary sources</u>:

Cereals & Millets	magnesium / 100 gm
Amaranth seeds	2 70 mg
Bajra	124 mg
Raagi	146 mg
Wheat flour, atta	125 mg
Jowar	133 mg

Grains and Legumes	magnesium / 100 gm
Horse gram	152 mg
Soya beans	259 mg
Bengal gram, whole	160 mg
Rajmah	173 mg
Black gram, dal	173 mg
Cow pea	213 mg
Field beans	173 mg
Green gram	198 mg
Peas, dry	123 mg
Red gram	119 mg

Green leafy vegetables	magnesium / 100 gm
Amranth leaves, green	194 mg
Basella leaves	153 mg
Amranth leaves, red	177 mg
Betel leaves	107 mg
Beet green	120 mg

Nuts & Oil seeds	Magnesium / 100 gm
Gingelly seeds, black	390 mg
Gingelly seeds, white	372 mg
Niger seeds, black	346 mg
Mustard seeds	266 mg
Garden cress seeds	307 mg
Lin seeds	349 mg
Almonds	318 mg
Safflower seeds	321 mg
Sunflower seeds	413 mg
Pistachio nuts	149 mg
Walnut	180 mg
Ground nuts	197 mg
Cashew nuts	307 mg
Pine seeds	268 mg

Sugars	Magnesium / 100 gm
Jaggery, cane	115 mg

Phosphorus

Phosphorus is an important non metallic constituent. The amount of phosphorous in the body exceed only by calcium, in bones the proportion of calcium to phosphorus is about 2:1 ration. The proportion of phosphorous in body fluids & soft tissue is much higher than calcium.

Functions of Phosphorous:

- Essential to our health, most abundant mineral.
- Important for formation & maintenance of
  - o Bone, teeth health.
  - o Helps kidneys to filter wastes.
  - o Energy production, storage.
  - o Growth, maintenance, tissue repair.
  - o Formation of nucleic acid for cell division, DNA & RNA synthesis.
  - o Maintains healthy levels of Vit. D, Calcium, Iodine, Magnesium, Zinc.
  - o Acid- base balance.

o It is needed for milk secretion (Lactation)

Deficiency Symptoms:

- Lack of Phosphorous leads to weakness, loss of weight, bone density, appetite, osteoporosis, muscle control, muscle strength, trembling, convulsion, high blood pressure, arteriosclerosis & heart disease.
- Problems associated with respiratory & central nervous system are also seen.

Recommended Dietary Allowance RDA of Phosphorous: is about 1gm/day.

Dietary sources:

- Phosphorous is present mostly in all foods but particularly high in protein rich foods, such as dairy, pulses as well as green leafy vegetables & in most fruits.

Cereals & Millets	Phosphorous / 100 gm
Amaranth seeds	0.4 gm
Bajra	0.2 gm
Raagi	0.2 gm
Wheat flour, atta	0.3 gm
Jowar	0.2 gm

Grains and Legumes	Phosphorous / 100 gm
Horse gram	0.2 gm
Soya beans	0.4 gm
Bengal gram, whole	0.2 gm
Rajmah	0.4 gm
Black gram, dal	0.3 gm
Cow pea	0.3 gm
Field beans	0.4 gm
Green gram	0.4 gm
Peas, dry	0.3 gm
Red gram	0.3 gm

Milk and Milk products	Phosphorous / 100 gm
Koha	0.4 gm
Panner	0.3 gm

Egg & Egg Products	Phosphorous / 100 gm
Egg, poultry, yolk, boiled	0.5 gm
Egg, poultry, whole, boiled	0.2 gm

Copper

Copper is widely distributed in the body about 95% is found in blood plasma (firmly bond by a protein complex). The highest amount of copper is found in brain & liver tissue. Zinc and Vitamin C supplements are strong antagonists of copper absorptions. Most of the copper is excreted through bile in faecal matter.

Functions:

- Copper helps in the metabolism of iron, glucose & protein.
- Helps in production of RBC's.
- Growth & development of bone, connective tissue and brain.
- Stimulate immune system, promotes healing.
- Act as antioxidant, helps in nerve cell function.
- Prevents anemia, osteoporosis, cardio vascular disease, Alzheimer's disease.
- Copper helps in the manufacturing of thyroid-stimulating hormone. And also insulation of myelin sheet around the nerves.

Deficiency symptoms:

- Anemia, Hair problems, dry skin, general weakness, low body temperature, bone fracture, osteoporosis, atherosclerosis, irregular heartbeat, digestive problems, thyroid problems.
- Other symptoms are high blood pressure, kidney disease, signs of early aging.

Causes of copper deficiency:

- High dose of Zinc supplement causes copper deficiency, as copper and zinc is strong antagonist in nature, so deficiency in zinc increase copper absorption. An excess of copper causes Zinc loss. Vitamin C supplements are strong antagonist of copper absorption.

Recommended Dietary Allowance RDA of Copper: is about 2mg/day.

Dietary sources:

Copper deficiency is uncommon. Even poor diet provide enough copper for human needs.

Nuts & Oil seeds	Copper / 100 gm
Gingelly seeds, black	1.76mg
Gingelly seeds, white	1.50mg
Niger seeds, black	1.20 mg
Lin seeds	1.34 mg
Almonds	1.08mg
Sunflower seeds	2.78 mg
Walnut	1.52 mg
Cashew nuts	2.23mg
Pine seeds	1.17mg

Grains and Legumes	Copper / 100 gm
Horse gram	1.29 mg
Soya beans	1.29 mg
Field beans	1.03 mg
Green gram	1.0 mg
Red gram	1.14 mg

Fluorine

Fluorine is a trace element found in great variety of foods, in very small amount. Traces of fluorine are found in bones, teeth, thyroid gland & skin. It protects teeth form decay.

Functions:

- Fluorine is a mineral mainly found in teeth & skeleton.
- Helps to protect teeth & bones against decay.
- Consumed during childhood becomes a part of dental enamel, strengthens tooth greatly & reduce the chance of decay/ caries developing in the teeth.
- Make teeth & bone resistant to the weak organic acids.

Deficiency symptoms:

- Fluorine is often known as a two-edged sword. If the fluoride content of drinking water is below 0.5 PPM (Part per Million), increase more prevalence towards dental caries.

- Fluorine doesn't totally prevent dental caries, but it can reduce the prevalence by 60-70%.

Recommended Dietary Allowance RDA of Fluorine:

Fluoride is required in small amount. About 1 PPM (Part per Million) is considered enough for normal healthy teeth & bones.

Dietary source:

- The main source of fluorine for most human beings is the drinking water.
- If the water has fluorine content of about 1PPM then it will supply adequate fluorine for the teeth & bone.
- In addition the average diet may provide 0.25-0.35 mg of Fluorine.

Note:

- Soft water has little or no fluorine. Where in some developing countries they add fluoride to tooth paste also helps to reduce dental caries (but beware about the fluorine content it should not exceed the normal level. whereas not more than 1PPM.)
- While in hard water the fluorine content may be high as 6-10 PPM, and excessively high intake of fluoride causes a dental fluorosis, in which teeth become mottled. It also cause bone changes with selerosis (added bone density) leads to a condition called skeletal fluorosis which causes severe pain & serious bone abnormalities.

Iodine:

Iodine is required for growth & survival for human life. It is chiefly derived from the ocean & the soil. About one-third of the iodine present in adults occur in the thyroid gland whereas about 25- 50 mg. The degree of absorption of iodine in the body depends upon the level of thyroid hormone circulating in the blood.

Functions:

- Iodine is essential for synthesis & metabolism of the thyroid hormone, thyroxin.
- It is a constitute of thyroid gland, which controls the rate of energy utilized in the body (BMR).
- Thyroxin helps to regulate the rate of oxidation within the cells which stimulate physical & mental growth, functioning of nerve &

muscle tissue growth, circulation of blood & metabolism of all nutrients required for the body.
- Iodine supports the brain function, without enough iodine the child could be mentally retarded.
- All cells in the body require iodine for their normal functioning, reproductive organs, breast, ovaries, prostate; testiciles all require iodine for their healthy functioning.
- Iodine helps in detoxification.
- Iodine helps to reduce the need for insulin, it involves in slowing down of diabetes, stabilizing the blood sugar.

Deficiency symptoms: (Iodine deficiency disorders:IDD's)

-Iodine deficiency can affect all age groups especially has great impact on fetus in the womb during pregnancy or in the period soon after birth, it affects the developing brain and physical growth of babies.

In the severe case of Iodine deficiency in a new born child can cause Cretinism, a condition characterized by several mental retardation, stunted growth, impaired speech, movement, hearing.

In Adults Deficiency of iodine causes goiter. Characterized by swelling of thyroid gland, the reduced secretion of thyroid gland can lead to several other problems in the body.

Other symptoms of iodine deficiency are obesity, swelling of thyroid gland (hypothyroid), saliva deficiency, brain feel sluggish, Morning sickness, mental retardation, fibrocystic breast, cyst in ovaries/testicles, prostate enlargement , PCOS, Hormonal imbalance (lot of menstrual issue) ,Miscarriages'/Still birth. Cancer to the breast, stomach and cancers can occurs

Causes of iodine deficiency:

-In the hilly area where there is deficiency of iodine in foods and drinking water (soil doesn't have enough amount of iodine in it).

-Eating more amount of cruciferous foods (cabbage, cauliflower), which have tendency to reduce iodine uptake.

-Eating low salt diet.

-Eating too much of soya (estrogenic) deplete iodine in body, affects thyroid.

-Endocrine disrupters like pesticides, vermicides, fungicides and even heavy metals like bromide, mercury, fluoride from food(processed foods like biscuits, breads etc..) or environment can also block the absorption of iodine.

-Stress-cortical (stress hormone) reduce the iodine absorption.

-Hormonal imbalance during pregnancy, hormonal replacement therapy, Birth control pills, high levels of estrogen, severely blocks the iodine receptor cells.

- Liver damage (low bile) or kidney damage can also cause iodine deficiency (Because, liver/gall bladder and kidney helps to convert inactive thyroid hormone to active form .

Recommended dietary allowance:

A teaspoon of iodine is all a person requires in a lifetime. However the thyroid gland does not have a capacity to store this amount of iodine in it so, small amount of iodine must be consumed regularly in the diet. The World health organization recommended the following daily intake for optimal iodine nutrition:

WHO daily intake : optimal iodine nutrition	
Population sub groups	Amount
Infants (0-5yrs)	90μg/day
Pregnancy and lactation	200μg/day
Children (6-12yrs)	120μg/day
Adults	150μg/day

Dietary source:

The richest food source for iodine is sea foods(Tuna, salmon), because ocean is a big reservoir of iodine. The iodine levels in food of animal origin are higher than plant origin. The iodine is generally supplied by food and water, provided the soil contains in it.

Iodine rich foods are egg, meat, dairy products (milk, curd), Iodine rich of Plant origin are potato, green leafy vegetables (spinach),legumes, peas, beans, etc..

REFERENCES

1. C. Gopalan, T. Longvah, R. Ananthan, K. Bhaskarachary, K. Venkaiah, 2017, Indian Food Comosition Tables. National Institute of Nutrition, Indian Council of medical Research, Hyderabad.

2. Vinodini Reddy, K. Vijayaraghavan, 1995, Carotene rich foods for combating vitamin A Deficiency. National Institute of Nutrition, Indian Council of medical Research, Hyderabad.

3. P.S. Venkatachalam, L.M. Rebello, Reprinted: 2004, 2011, Nutrition for Mother and Child. National Institute of Nutrition, Indian Council of medical Research, Hyderabad.

4. A Manual, Dietary Guidelines for Indians, Second Edition: 2011, National Institute of Nutrition, Indian Council of medical Research, Hyderabad.

5. Jyoti singh, 2012, Hand book of Nutrition & Dietetics